Instructor's Guide for

Diseases of the Human Body
3rd edition

Carol D. Tamparo, PhD, CMA-A
Dean, Business and Allied Health
Lake Washington Technical College
Kirkland, Washington

Marcia A. Lewis, EdD, RN, CMA-AC
Associate Dean, Mathematics, Engineering Sciences, and Health
Adjunct Instructor, Medical Assisting
Olympic College
Bremerton, Washington

With contributions by

Marty Hitchcock, AS, CMA
Program Director, Medical Assisting
Gwinnett Technical Institute
Lawrenceville, Georgia

Valerie Nye, LPN, BSEd, CMA
Medical Assistant Program Director
Lake Washington Technical College
Kirkland, Washington

Carol Cassell, BS, RN, Health Educator
Associate Faculty Member
Department of Medical Assisting
Consumnes River Community College
Sacramento, California

F. A. Davis Company
1915 Arch Street
Philadelphia, PA 19103

Printed in the United States of America

Last digit indicates print number: 10 9 8 7 6 5 4 3 2 1

Publisher: Jean-François Vilain
Senior Editor: Lynn Borders Caldwell
Developmental Editors: Christa Fratantoro & Julia M. Catagnus
Cover Designer: Louis Forgione

ISBN 0-8036-0565-X

CONTENTS

INTRODUCTION

Class presentations on the topic of diseases may be one of your greatest challenges. You will be called upon to share your knowledge of the subject with the benefit of limited demonstration activities.

Since students' learning patterns are aural, visual, or activity oriented, the success of your class presentations may depend upon your ability to use as many of these modalities as possible to describe a particular disease well enough to assist students in their learning.

Critical Thinking

There will be no better opportunity for you to teach and encourage critical thinking skills than in this class. Critical thinking is the process used to encourage students to synthesize the information, assimilate the material, and be able to make valid assumptions and to draw conclusions. Critical thinking is experiential learning that requires students to be actively involved.

For example, when considering acute appendicitis, ask students what might cause such a condition. Students should be able to identify at least one or two causes. Using these responses, carry their thinking a step further into a discussion of possible symptoms that may or may not be indicative of appendicitis. If a client shares these symptoms on the phone, what questions will you ask? What diagnostic procedures will be necessary to determine a diagnosis? Soon, without being fully aware of the process, students will have been required to think critically about appendicitis and will have obtained the essential knowledge.

Your role as instructor will be to ask questions and facilitate students' thinking, sometimes fogging the issue, and always encouraging students to clarify and analyze the facts given.

Guest Lecturers

If verbal presentations are not your best mode of teaching (instructors, like students, have preferences when it comes to learning methods), you will want to use as many outside presenters as possible.

Physicians, nurses, or individuals suffering from a particular disease are better able to describe a disease process than is someone who has no firsthand experience.

Guest lecturers serve the class needs best when they have prior knowledge of your expectations. For example, if you ask a dermatologist to speak about diseases of the skin, the following outline may prove helpful:

1) Explain the educational background needed to become a dermatologist.
2) Discuss the types of referrals you receive.
3) Discuss the more common diseases of the skin.
4) Describe some common diagnostic procedures you use.
5) Define preventive measures we can take.

Also, it is helpful to inform the guest about the previous courses students have completed, the information you have covered in this class, and the diseases in their specialty area that are described in *Diseases of the Human Body*.

Your Personal Development

As a means of furthering your own professional development, it may be helpful to seek permission from a hospital to view several autopsies. Immersing yourself in advanced pathology texts will also provide access to photographs, illustrations, and information beyond those presented in *Diseases of the Human Body.* Use the Internet to download information, photographs, and illustrations for use in class. You may also find it beneficial to use the computer in class to demonstrate its use as well as to teach students about specific diseases. Your most helpful resources will generally come from widely known and respected sources. Remember to use caution in presenting any outside references in order to ensure their accuracy. The more you are able to provide students with materials not already presented in the text, the more comfortable you will feel in class.

For some diseases, vast amounts of material are available for your use. For example, contacting the American Cancer Society will bring you pamphlets, booklets, films, and even a list of potential guest lecturers. See the Appendices for names and addresses of additional organizations.

Teaching Strategies

Students who are personally affected by a disease you are discussing, or know someone who is, will be your strongest allies or your worst enemies. Ask during the first week of class if any students wish to research a specific disease. You may want to schedule these presentations with a time limit and suggest that students provide a one page summary so that copies can be distributed to the class.

Some students will be convinced at some time during the class that they have all the symptoms you are describing and are likely to die before the class is finished. They may ask you for medical advice. Some students may indeed have the diseases you are discussing. Whether or not this is true, you must temper your remarks with caution. Be candid. Keep in mind the needs of persons who may be suffering these diseases. You must refrain from practicing medicine or giving medical advice. Remind students of the same as some may tend to feel powerful with even limited information. It is better to encourage respect for the unknown and the authority of those with more knowledge.

Because you cannot be expected to know all the answers to the questions you may be asked, "I don't know" is a good and honest response. You may be able to find the answer, to ask the student to research the question, or redirect the class to the original topic of discussion with no additional input.

Diseases of the Human Body uses a format of presentation based on the knowledge most useful for health-care professionals in their actual work environment. It would be useful for you to explain to students how this format will be used in the actual work setting. The description of a disease and a few signs and symptoms are most likely the first information coming from the patient via the telephone or in person. The etiology of a disease together with signs and symptoms will help determine the diagnostic procedures performed. Health-care professionals must understand treatment since it is of paramount importance to the person. The prognosis and prevention are an important part of the ongoing education process.

Customizing the Book for Your Course

The best teaching and learning on the subject of diseases occurs when students already have a basic understanding of medical terminology, human anatomy, and physiology. In some programs these courses are taught in an integrated manner while in others the diseases class is designed to stand alone. In either instance, the diseases class is best presented after the student has a conceptual knowledge of medical terminology, anatomy, and physiology. If an anatomy and physiology or medical terminology text is used in conjunction with the teaching of diseases, the recommendation is to select those chapter topics that coincide and to include the remainder of the disease chapters as time permits.

You may choose to eliminate some chapters from the text. Chapters that are shorter in length ("Neoplasms," "Pain and Its Management," and "The Holistic Approach to Disease") may be combined with other more lengthy chapters.

Suggestions for Student Assignments

1) Have each student select a disease not included in the text or one that is very briefly described, and have the student write a five to seven page research paper on that disease entity. An oral report to the class could be included as part of the assignment or as a separate one.
2) Have students identify individuals who have a disease described in the text and interview them to see if the individual "fits" the clinical picture presented. Have students report on how the individual's experience differs from that described in the text.
3) Encourage students to check the educational channels on television for disease-related programs. Often surgical techniques and diagnostic procedures are pictured and discussed. A report could then be made to the class.

Audiovisual Aids

Audiovisual aids are essential in teaching *Diseases of the Human Body*. Researching the library for such resources is your first step. A computer search of your library's resources may be all you need or you may need to request some audiovisual materials through interlibrary loan. A useful resource is:

Films for the Humanities & Sciences, Inc.
P.O. Box 2053
Princeton, NJ 08543-2053
1-800-257-5126 or 609-452-1128
Fax 609-275-3767
8:30 AM to 5:30 PM Eastern Time

Additionally, the authors recommend that you keep a blank videotape close to your television and VCR to record programs about diseases, diagnostic procedures, surgeries, and disease prevention. Encourage students to do the same. New technologies and treatments are developed almost daily. Such a videotape could be viewed in class and then discussed. Be aware of any copyright requirements.

Researching Diseases on the Internet

The following is a description of the process for accessing information on the Internet, using *carpal tunnel syndrome* as an example:

Using an Internet browser program, go to the icon labeled *Search* at the top center of the program's icon bar. Click once. Then choose any of the Internet search engines (e.g., Lycos, Excite, Infoseek, Yahoo, Web Crawler, or Alta Vista) by clicking on the appropriate button. Key in the words *carpal tunnel syndrome*. Click on the button nearest to the word labeled *Search* or *Go to*. The search engine will search the Internet to find Web sites including information about carpal tunnel syndrome. Each site will then be listed, along with a brief description of the site and the address for accessing it.

A faster and more targeted method is to click on the word *health* at the Internet guide general information directory. At the *health* site you will be able to choose from the topics listed or search for more specific topics by keying them in at the site.

Examples of sites to look at are: http://www.sechrest.com/nmg/cts/ctsintro.html
http://www.phys.com
http://www.netaxs.com/people/iris/cts/

Keying in any of the above addresses on the site/address line at the top of the browser program will take you directly to the site. Otherwise, just pick a topic and search the Internet until you find a site that interests you. At anytime you can use the *Back, Forward*, or *Home* icons at the center Internet icon bar to return to a familiar site of the original site.

Expect to work hard and learn much preparing for this class. Medicine is ever growing. What we know of the disease process is being expanded and modified daily. If you enter into the experience with enthusiasm, it will be contagious. There is no greater joy than teaching enthusiastic students.

Suggested Course Schedule For A 10-Week Quarter

Week	Chapter in Text
1	1. The Disease Process
2	2. Infectious Diseases 4. Congenital Diseases
3	3. Neoplasms 15. Pain and its Management 16. The Holistic Approach to Disease
4	5. Urinary System Diseases 6. Reproductive System Diseases
5	6. Reproductive System Diseases—continued 7. Digestive System Diseases
6	8. Respiratory System Diseases
7	9. Circulatory System Diseases
8	10. Nervous System Diseases
9	11. Endocrine System Diseases 12. Musculoskeletal Diseases
10	13. Skin Diseases 14. Eye and Ear Diseases

Suggested Course Schedule For A 16-Week Semester

Week	Chapter in Text
1	1. The Disease Process
2	2. Infectious Diseases
3	3. Neoplasms
4	4. Congenital Diseases
5	5. Urinary System Diseases
6	6. Reproductive System Diseases
7	7. Digestive System Diseases
8	8. Respiratory System Diseases
9	9. Circulatory System Diseases
10	10. Nervous System Diseases
11	11. Endocrine System Diseases
12	12. Musculoskeletal Diseases
13	13. Skin Diseases
14	14. Eye and Ear Diseases
15	15. Pain and its Management
16	16. The Holistic Approach to Disease

CHAPTER 1: THE DISEASE PROCESS

Chapter Goal

To introduce students to the disease process.

Learning Objectives

Upon successful completion of the chapter and class lecture and discussion, students will respond to the following on a written exam within the allotted class time with a minimum of ____% accuracy.

- Define disease.
- Contrast illness and disease.
- Restate at least three predisposing factors of disease.
- Identify the three classifications of hereditary diseases.
- Describe DNA's genetic activity.
- Distinguish between genotype and phenotype.
- Identify the process of inflammation.
- Describe how infections are transmitted.
- Name at least four groups of microorganisms.
- Identify the most likely anatomic sites for traumatic injuries.
- Recall at least six chemical agents/irritants that may cause disease.
- Contrast neoplasm and cancer.
- Define benign and malignant tumors.
- Identify three means of protection afforded by the immune system.
- Differentiate between
    - Natural and acquired immunity.
    - Humoral and cell-mediated immunity.
    - B-cell and T-cell immunity.
- Name three classifications of immune-related diseases.
- Identify a disease associated with each type of allergy.
- Describe how anaphylactic shock can occur in any of the allergic reactions.
- Name four categories of immunodeficiency diseases.
- Explain mental and emotional factors as a cause of illness.
- Give three examples of nutritional imbalance.
- Define idiopathic and iatrogenic diseases.

Class Activities

Having a solid base of understanding of the disease process will make it easier for students to comprehend other chapters. There are some basic principles related to the cause of disease that all students should know. It is important to discuss the difference between illness and disease. Predisposing factors should be considered, also.

The most challenging areas to present to students are the sections on hereditary diseases and immune-related factors. Keep the discussion at a level appropriate for students to comprehend. Keep in mind that students coming into your classes with little or no education in science and biology may have particular difficulty.

It is important to establish the parameters for your class during these early sessions. If you wish to have students prepare a report on a specific disease, this is the time to introduce the concept and make assignments. An interesting method of beginning the discussion of this chapter is to ask each student to identify his or her most recent illness. List these on the board and as you discuss the disease process, relate it to these illnesses. This will help students remember the disease process is varied, complex, and sometimes has multiple causes.

Test Questions

Chapter 1: The Disease Process

CIRCLE THE ONE BEST ANSWER.

1. Factors influencing the disease process in the elderly include
a. Psychological changes.
b. Decreased immunity.
c. Degenerative conditions.
d. Both b and c

2. Phenotype is a word used to describe
a. Inherited diseases.
b. Physical appearance.
c. Body build.
d. Color vision.

3. Hemophilia is a/an
a. Multifactorial disorder.
b. Chromosomal disorder.
c. X or sex-linked disorder.
d. Autosomal disorder.

4. Diseases caused by bacteria include
a. Diphtheria.
b. Yellow fever.
c. Hepatitis.
d. Rocky Mountain Spotted Fever.

5. A predisposing factor
a. May make a person more susceptible to disease.
b. Might be age, gender, heredity, or environment.
c. a and b
d. All of the above.

6. Hereditary diseases
a. Always appear at birth.
b. May go undetected until adolescence or adulthood.
c. Are caused by a person's genetic makeup.
d. b and c

7. Anaphylactic shock is
a. Considered an allergic reaction.
b. A neoplastic malignancy of the lymph system.

c. Chronic and not life threatening.

d. Emotional or mental in etiology.

8. Obesity

a. Has been defined as being 10 to 20 percent above ideal body weight.

b. May be caused by too many calories or too little activity.

c. May be an endocrine or metabolic problem.

d. All of the above

9. The conventional method of classifying hereditary diseases is to group them into which of the following categories?

a. Congenital, mutational, and infectious

b. Chromosomal, multifactorial, and monogenic

c. Monogenic, chromosomal, and congenital

d. Chromosomal, mutational, and autoimmune

10. Environmental hazards that may have an effect on health might include

a. Pollutants such as car exhaust and loud noise.

b. Geographical location.

c. Heavy computer use.

d. All of the above

11. Which of the following conditions IS NOT a genetic disorder?

a. Cystic fibrosis

b. Sickle cell anemia

c. Carpal tunnel syndrome

d. Phenylketonuria

12. The body's response to physical trauma, chemical agents, infections, and allergies is inflammation, which includes

a. Redness, pain, and loss of function.

b. Heat, swelling, and loss of function.

c. Redness, pain, swelling, and loss of function.

d. Redness, heat, pain, swelling, and loss of function.

13. The leading cause of death in the United States for persons younger than 35 is

a. Infection.

b. Hereditary disease.

c. Trauma.

d. Chemical exposure.

14. The leading cause of death in young children is

a. Asphyxiation.

b. Near-drowning.

c. Poisoning.

d. Burns.

15. An idiopathic disease

a. Is transmitted genetically.

4

b. Has no known cause.
c. Is caused by medical treatment.
d. Is caused by trauma.

16. An iatrogenic disease
a. Is transmitted genetically.
b. Has no known cause.
c. Is caused by medical treatment.
d. Is caused by trauma.

17. The "rule of nines" can be used to assess the extent/severity of
a. Hereditary diseases.
b. Near-drownings.
c. Burns.
d. Infections.

18. Which of the following microorganisms include yeasts and molds?
a. Fungi
b. Rickettsiae
c. Protozoa
d. Viruses

19. The large division of worm-like internal parasites is
a. Rhizopus.
b. Aspergillus.
c. Helminths.
d. Plasmodium.

20. The smallest parasitic microorganisms are
a. Bacilli.
b. Cocci.
c. Tapeworms.
d. Viruses.

21. The leading cause of death in the United States for persons younger than 35 years of age is
a. Viral infections.
b. Cancer.
c. Physical trauma.
d. Asphyxiation.

22. Brain tissue is bruised and normal nerve function is disrupted by
a. Frostbite.
b. Contusions.
c. Concussions.
d. Skull fractures.

23. Extreme cold may cause
a. Chilblain.

b. Hypothermia.
c. Hypovolemic shock.
d. a and b

24. Which of the following causes a lack of oxygen and accumulation of carbon dioxide in the blood?
a. Electric shock
b. Poisoning
c. Asphyxiation
d. Neoplasia

25. Which of the following is classified by extent, depth, client age, and associated illness and injury?
a. Insect, snake, and spider bites
b. Burns
c. Allergies
d. Physical trauma

26. The spreading process of a malignant tumor or cancer is
a. Tachycardia.
b. Sarcoma.
c. In situ.
d. Metastasis.

27. The action by a group of white cells called T-cell lymphocytes is
a. Cell-mediated immunity.
b. Humoral immunity.
c. Phagocytosis.
d. Lymphadenopathy.

28. Chemical or physical agents/irritants that may cause disease are
a. Extremes of atmospheric pressure.
b. Poisoning and ionizing radiation.
c. Allergies and eczema.
d. a and b

29. Which of the following is not true about DNA's genetic activity?
a. The DNA is a complex molecular structure in the cell nucleus that is incorporated into chromosomes.
b. At the time of fertilization, the 23 chromosomes from the ovum combine randomly with the same number from the sperm.
c. Dominant genes are expressed only when the gene pair is homozygous, whereas recessive genes are expressed whether the gene pair is homozygous or heterozygous.
d. Mutations that occur when the normal sequence of DNA units is disrupted can cause functional disturbances in the body.

30. Illness differs from disease in that illness
a. Encompasses how individuals perceive themselves as suffering from a disease.
b. Is easier for health-care providers to treat.

c. Is known by its medical classification and distinguishing features.
d. All of the above

31. Inflammation is defined as
a. The body's response to trauma, physical or chemical agents, and pathogenic organisms.
b. Being acute or chronic.
c. A process beginning with the physical irritant and ending with healing.
d. All of the above

32. Included in the groups classified as microorganisms are
a. Fungi and parasites.
b. Rickettsiae and protozoa.
c. Bacteria and viruses.
d. All of the above.

DEFINE

33. Idiopathic:

34. Iatrogenic:

35. Benign Tumors:

36. Malignant Tumor:

Answers

Chapter 1: The Disease Process

1. d (p. 3)

2. b (p. 4)

3. c (p. 6)

4. a (p. 8)

5. c (p. 3)

6. d (p. 3-4)

7. a (p. 16)

8. d (p. 18)

9. b (p. 4)

10. d (p. 3)

11. c (p. 3-4)

12. d (p. 6)

13. c (p. 9-10)

14. d (p. 13)

15. b (p. 19)

16. c (p. 19)

17. c (p. 13-14)

18. a (p. 7)

19. c (p. 9)

20. d (p. 8)

21. c (p.9)

22. b (p. 10)

23. d (p. 12)

24. c (p. 13)

25. b (p. 15)

26. d (p. 13)

27. a (p. 15)

28. d (p. 11)

29. c (p. 4)

30. a (p. 3)

31. d (p. 6)

32. d (p. 7-9)

33. disease having no known cause (p. 19)

34. caused by treatment and its effects in patients (p. 19)

35. new formation or growth that remains circumscribed, although it may vary in size (p. 13)

36. cancer that spreads to other cell tissues, and parts of the body through the bloodstream or lymphatic system (p. 13)

CHAPTER 2: INFECTIOUS DISEASES

Chapter Goal

To acquaint students with the description, etiology, signs and symptoms, diagnostic procedures, treatment, prognosis, and prevention of the most common infectious diseases.

Learning Objectives

Upon successful completion of the chapter and class lecture and discussion, students will respond to the following on a written exam within the allotted class time with a minimum of ____% accuracy.

- Recall the symptoms of colds.
- Describe the treatment of influenza.
- Define chronic fatigue syndrome.
- Restate at least six signs or symptoms of chronic fatigue syndrome.
- Discuss the etiology of AIDS.
- Recall the prevention of AIDS.
- Identify the etiology and three stages of Lyme disease.
- Discuss the foodborne infection *Escherichia Coli* 0157:H7.
- List the most common communicable diseases of childhood and adolescence.
- Recall the signs and symptoms of measles.
- Distinguish between measles and rubella.
- Identify the classic symptoms of mumps.
- Describe the treatment of varicella.
- Explain measures to prevent diphtheria.
- Discuss the two stages of pertussis.
- Describe the signs and symptoms of tetanus.

Class Activities

Students will have a fair amount of knowledge of infectious diseases. There are volumes of information available for the lay person that describe the infectious process and offer advice on prevention. A fair amount of misinformation and lack of awareness of the unusual or unexpected exceptions to the infectious disease process may accompany this knowledge, information, and experience.

The information is constantly changing and being expanded. The media continually addresses warnings related to cooking, handling, and storage of food and beverage. In addition, the overuse of antibiotics has caused some infectious diseases to become increasingly resistant to treatment.

Consider inviting a speaker from the county health department or a community health nurse who can bring information about the most common infectious diseases and the alarming changes in patterns of infectious disease. Since you will find many childhood diseases addressed in this chapter, you may want to seek the advice of a pediatrician.

Teaching communicable diseases of childhood and adolescence may be difficult for students and teacher alike, especially if many audiovisual aides are used. No one likes to hear about or visualize an ill child or young person.

Another difficult area to teach in this chapter is the description of communicable diseases, especially if you or your students have never seen the effects of such diseases. More in-depth pathology texts and Internet sites contain illustrations and photographs that may prove helpful.

Name_____

Test Questions

    Chapter 2: Infectious Diseases

CIRCLE THE ONE BEST ANSWER:

1. HIV can be transmitted through
a. Saliva.
b. Nasal secretions.
c. Air droplets.
d. Blood and blood products

2. Influenza is spread through
a. Respiratory droplets.
b. Objects contaminated with discharge.
c. Air droplets from sneeze or cough.
d. All of the above

3. The most common pulmonary infection associated with AIDS is
a. *Pneumocystis carinii* pneumonia.
b. Bronchitis.
c. *Pneumococcal* pneumonia.
d. *Streptococcal* pneumonia .

4. The white blood cells that are affected the most by HIV are
a. Monocytes.
b. Eosinophils.
c. Lymphocytes.
d. Neutrophils.

5. The specific *Escherichia coli* bacteria that has been causing serious illness is being spread by
a. Sewage-contaminated water.
b. Undercooked meat products.
c. Pasteurized milk and fruit juices.
d. a and b

6. The incubation period for pertussis is
a. 5 days.
b. 14 days.
c. 15 to 20 days.
d. 7 to 10 days.

7. A vaccine is a
a. Suspension of living infectious agents and a solution of toxins from microorganisms.

b. Solution of toxins from microorganisms and a solution of a nonpathogen.

c. Suspension of living infectious agents and a solution of a nonpathogen.

d. Solution of a nonpathogen.

8. Which of the following communicable diseases exhibits Koplik's spots on the oral mucosa?

a. Rubeola

b. Rubella

c. Mumps

d. Varicella

9. Another name for German measles is

a. Rubeola.

b. Rubella.

c. Varicella.

d. Pertussis.

10. Which of the following diseases has the classic symptom of unilateral or bilateral swollen parotid glands?

a. Diphtheria

b. Varicella

c. Mumps

d. Tetanus

11. Another name for pertussis is

a. Lockjaw.

b. Chickenpox.

c. Measles.

d. Whooping cough.

12. A highly contagious disease with a distinctive rash that passes through stages of muscles, papules, vesicles, and crusts is called

a. Influenza.

b. Tetanus.

c. Pertussis.

d. Varicella.

13. An acute, life-threatening infectious disease characterized by a membranelike coating that forms over mucous membrane surfaces, especially the respiratory tract, is known as

a. Diphtheria.

b. Mumps.

c. Influenza.

d. Varicella.

14. An acute, highly infectious respiratory tract disease characterized by a repetitious, paroxysmal cough and a prolonged, harsh or shrill sound during inspiration is called

a. Tetanus.

b. Bronchitis.

c. Laryngitis.
d. Pertussis.

15. Tetanus is caused by a bacterium commonly found in
a. Soil.
b. Food.
c. The gastrointestinal tract.
d. Human tissue.

16. The U.S. Public Health Service recommends inoculation against influenza for which
of the following groups of people?
a. The elderly, individuals with serious systemic disease, and individuals with chronic respiratory disease
b. The elderly and individuals with chronic respiratory disease
c. Individuals with serious system disease and children
d. Children only

17. Varicella treatment consists of
a. Isolation.
b. Calamine lotion.
c. Bicarbonate of soda baths.
d. All of the above

18. Signs and symptoms of tetanus include
a. Stiffness of esophageal muscles.
b. Severe convulsive muscle spasms.
c. Painful lymph nodes.
d. a and b only

19. The 0157:H7 strain of *Escherichia coli*
a. Lives in the intestinal tract of humans.
b. Is an emerging cause of food-borne illness.
c. Causes constipation and respiratory distress.
d. a only

20. A viral respiratory infection that may be prevented by immunization is
a. The common cold.
b. Influenza.
c. Chronic fatigue syndrome.
d. Acquired immune deficiency syndrome.

21. The treatment of influenza includes
a. Antibiotics, bedrest, adequate fluid intake, and antipyretics.
b. Bedrest and adequate fluid intake only,
c. Antibiotics, adequate fluid intake, and antipyretics.
d. Bedrest, adequate fluid intake, and antipyretics.

22. A condition with an unknown etiology characterized by sudden prolonged,
unbearable exhaustion with the following associated symptoms: fever, nonexudative

pharyngitis, arthralgia, photophobia, and unexplained muscle weakness can be symptoms of which disease?

a. Influenza

b. Chronic fatigue syndrome

c. Rubella

d. Acquired immune deficiency syndrome

23. Symptoms of the common cold include

a. Joint and muscle pain.

b. Nasal congestion and pharyngitis.

c. Headache, burning/watery eyes, and low-grade fever.

d. b and c

24. Signs and symptoms of chronic fatigue syndrome include

a. Muscle weakness and myalgia.

b. Photophobia and forgetfulness.

c. Sleep disturbance and transient visual scotomata.

d. a and b

25. In stage I of Lyme disease,

a. Diagnosis is fairly easy to establish.

b. Flulike symptoms may be the only evidence of the disease.

c. ECM rash is usually present.

d. Symptoms are constant and unchanging.

26. Diagnosis of Lyme disease during stage II or III can be made by

a. An abnormally high ESR.

b. An elevated total serum IgM level.

c. An increased aspartate aminotransferase level.

d. All of the above

Answers

Chapter 2: Infectious Diseases

1. d (p. 30)

2. d (p. 31)

3. a (p. 31)

4. c (p. 30)

5. d (p. 33)

6. a (p. 39)

7. a (p. 33-34)

8. a (p. 34)

9. b (p. 34)

10. c (p. 37)

11. d (p. 39)

12. d (p. 37)

13. a (p. 38)

14. d (p. 39)

15. a (p. 40)

16. a (p. 29)

17. d (p. 37)

18. d (p. 40)

19. d (p. 32-33)

20. b (p. 29)

21. d (p. 29)

22. b (p. 30)

23. d (p. 28-29)

24. c (p. 30)

25. b (p. 32)

26. d   (p. 32)

CHAPTER 3: NEOPLASMS

Chapter Goal

To acquaint students with neoplasms and cancerous growths and their risk factors and preventive measures.

Learning Objectives

Upon successful completion of the chapter and class lecture and discussion, students will respond to the following on a written exam within the allotted class time with a minimum of ____% accuracy:

- Define neoplasm.
- Compare benign and malignant tumors.
- Recall death statistics related to cancer.
- Identify at least eight suggestions for cancer prevention.
- List the seven warning signals of cancer.
- Describe the three main classifications of cancer.
- Identify the grading and staging of neoplasms and their use.
- List at least four possible causes of cancer.
- Discuss four major forms of cancer treatment and their advantages and disadvantages.
- Describe circumstances in which a physician and client may choose a combination of the four major cancer treatments.

Class Activities

A clear understanding of the medical terminology in this chapter is essential; otherwise, students may think all tumors are cancerous. Clarifying the differences between benign and malignant tumors is especially helpful. Take some time in class to discuss any concerns students have in this regard. You will also want to spend some time discussing the cancer risk factors, as well as preventive measures.

New research related to cancer, its incidence, and prevention is made public almost daily. Take advantage of this information for your class. You will want to visit the American Cancer Society in your area or search their site on the Internet. The volume of materials this organization has available for classroom use is far too great to detail here. They have a vast number of pamphlets, films, even models (e.g., breast models revealing varying sizes of lump), available for use. Also, they are usually able to supply speakers for your class who are willing to help make your study of neoplasms interesting, as well as informative. Consider asking a person with cancer to "tell his or her story." There is no one better able to describe what cancer does to a person, than someone who has lived with or is living with the illness.

The American Cancer Society can also supply you with the latest data related to incidence of the disease, since it is difficult for even a current textbook to be completely up-to-date. An oncologist in your area who can speak about the latest developments in cancer treatment would be another helpful and informative resource.

Name_____

Test Questions

Chapter 3: Neoplasms

CIRCLE THE ONE BEST ANSWER.

1. The main difference(s) between a malignant and a benign tumor is/are that the benign tumor
a. Is encapsulated.
b. Grows slowly.
c. Has the ability to spread into other parts of the body.
d. a and b

2. A measure to prevent cancer is to
a. Avoid red meat.
b. Eat plenty of fatty foods.
c. Avoid heavily polluted air.
d. a and c

3. Cancer cells go through several stages of growth, including
a. Hyperplasia.
b. Dysplasia.
c. Carcinoma in situ.
d. All of the above

4. Alternative treatment for cancer includes
a. Hormone therapy.
b. Radiation therapy.
c. Antineoplastic therapy.
d. Biotherapy.

5. Radiation therapy for cancer
a. Is received by about half of all persons with cancer.
b. May be used alone or in combination with other treatments.
c. Has little or no side affects.
d. a and b only

6. Common diagnostic procedures for cancer include
a. Breast exam and mammogram.
b. Pap test.
c. Prostate, rectal, and stool exams.
d. All the above

7. Grading and staging of neoplasms
a. Was developed by the American Cancer Society.
b. Is determined by microscopic appearance and the extent to which the tumor has spread.

c. Is done using four grades and the TNM system.
d. b and c only

8. Palliative surgery
a. Is done to sustain cancer patients and alleviate pain.
b. Prevents the development of cancer.
c. Freezes the malignancy.
d. a and c only

9. The term neoplasm may be used interchangeably with
a. Carcinogen.
b. Sarcoma.
c. Tumor.
d. Encapsulation.

10. An irreversible change in the structure of mature cells is referred to as
a. Differentiated.
b. Anaplastic.
c. In situ.
d. Blastic.

11. Neoplasms that closely resemble normal parent tissue are
a. Encapsulated.
b. Sarcomas.
c. Epithelial.
d. Differentiated.

12. A tumor that does not infiltrate surrounding tissue is
a. Metastasized.
b. Anaplastic.
c. Encapsulated.
d. Exfoliative.

13. A tumor that is in position, or localized, is
a. Anaplastic.
b. In situ.
c. Sarcoma.
d. Benign.

14. Removal of a small piece of living tissue for microscopic examination is
a. Biopsy
b. Cryosurgery.
c. Immunotherapy.
d. Radiation therapy.

15. Solid tumors of epithelial tissue of external and internal body surfaces are
a. Sarcomas.
b. Osteomas.
c. Leukemias.

d. Carcinomas.

16. A neoplasm that arises from the body's blood-forming tissues within the bone marrow is
a. Leukemia.
b. Lymphoma.
c. Sarcoma.
d. None of the above.

17. Tumors that arise from supportive and connective tissue are
a. In situ.
b. Carcinomas.
c. Sarcomas.
d. Leukemias.

18. A tumor that grows slowly and whose cells resemble normal cells of the tissue from which it originated is
a. Benign.
b. Anaplastic.
c. Choriocarcinoma.
d. a and c

19. The freezing of a malignancy with a liquid nitrogen probe is
a. Particle beam therapy.
b. Cryosurgery.
c. Radiation therapy
d. Chemotherapy.

20. Which is not an early warning signal of cancer?
a. Change in bowel or bladder habits
b. Temporary alopecia
c. Unusual bleeding or discharge
d. Thickening or lump in the breast or elsewhere

Answers

Chapter 3: Neoplasms

1. d (p. 44)

2. c (p. 47)

3. d (p. 49)

4. c (p. 51)

5. d (p. 50)

6. d (p. 49)

7. d (p. 48)

8. a (p. 50)

9. c (p. 44)

10. b (p. 44)

11. d (p. 48)

12. c (p. 44)

13. b (p. 49)

14. a (p. 49)

15. d (p. 47)

16. a (p. 47)

17. c (p. 47)

18. a (p. 44)

19. b (p. 50)

20. b (p. 49)

CHAPTER 4: CONGENITAL DISEASES

Chapter Goal

To introduce students to congenital diseases that are present at birth and brought about by genetic causes, nongenetic causes, or a combination of the two.

Learning Objectives

Upon successful completion of the chapter and class lecture and discussion, students will respond to the following on a written exam within the allotted class time with a minimum of _____% accuracy:

Describe the three types of cerebral palsy.
• Identify the signs and symptoms of spina bifida, meningocele, and myelomeningocele.
• Recall the diagnostic procedures used for hydrocephalus.
• Recall the etiology of pyloric stenosis.
• Discuss Hirschsprung's disease.
• Review the prevention of erythroblastosis fetalis.
• Compare and contrast the various congenital defects of the heart.
• Define cryptorchidism.
• Compare and contrast the congenital defects of the ureter, bladder, and urethra.
• List the four common forms of clubfoot.
• Recall the etiology of congenital hip dysplasia.
• Describe the signs and symptoms of cystic fibrosis.
• Restate the diagnostic procedures for phenylketonuria (PKU).

Class Activities

In relating this chapter to your students, it is important to remember that congenital diseases refer to those problems that are present at birth and brought about by genetic causes, nongenetic causes, or a combination of the two. They may or may not be detected at birth. This chapter may stand alone in its presentation or may be integrated into other chapters since it is organized by body systems.

Because there is so much to be learned about many of these diseases, your class may benefit from independent research done by students. Prior to the class session(s) in which congenital diseases will be presented, assign one disease or disorder to each student. It should be the student's responsibility to research the disease or disorder and present to the class, identifying the major components as illustrated in the text. This is one way of making certain that students are at least partially prepared for class. Also, the participating students are not apt to easily forget the disease or disorder for which they prepared a presentation.

If you use such a tactic in class, be certain to reward the students with points earned and/or a grade for the assignment. Time spent on such a task should be worthy of grading and comments from the instructor.

The Internet can be a source of pamphlets and up-to-date information on the diseases and disorders that are known to be the result of birth defects, much of which can be quite helpful. Many current magazines include articles about some of the diseases and how parents cope with children with congenital problems.

Name_____

Test Questions

  Chapter 4: Congenital Diseases

CIRCLE THE ONE BEST ANSWER.

1. The etiology of cerebral palsy includes
a. Genetic factors.
b. Maternal diabetes.
c. Exposure to a teratogen.
d. Maternal influenza.

2. If an infant begins projectile vomiting in the second to fourth month after birth, a physician might suspect
a. Pyloric stenosis.
b. Cardiac stenosis.
c. Hirschsprung's disease.
d. Cystic fibrosis.

3. Acyanotic heart defects in infants include
a. Coarctation of the aorta.
b. Tetralogy of Fallot.
c. Atrial septal defect.
d. a and c

4. The test to confirm cryptorchidism is
a. FSH.
b. Serum gonadotropin.
c. LH.
d. Serum testosterone .

5. Fatal complications of cystic fibrosis include
a. Shock.
b. Pneumonia.
c. Atelectasis.
d. All of the above

6. Cerebral palsy
a. Is bilateral, symmetrical, nonprogressive paralysis.
b. Results from developmental defects of the brain or trauma at birth.
c. a and b.
d. Diagnosis requires ultrasound examination for neural tube defects.

7. Neural tube defects
a. Almost always have an excellent prognosis without residual deficits.

b. Are characterized by hyperactive reflexes and rapid muscle contractions.

c. Require aggressive treatment without surgical intervention.

d. Are classified as spina bifida, meningocele, or myelomeningocele.

8. Hydrocephalus

a. Is a condition marked by too little cerebrospinal fluid in the ventricles of the brain.

b. May be classified as communicating or noncommunicating.

c. May be surgically treated with a shunt placed to drain excess fluid into venous circulation.

d. b and c

9. Hirschsprung's disease, or congenital aganglionic megacolon,

a. Is characterized by obstruction and dilation of the colon.

b. Is diagnosed by a rectal biopsy revealing the absence of ganglion cells in the colorectal wall.

c. May respond to surgery.

d. All of the above

10. Congenital cardiovascular diseases may include

a. Erythroblastosis fetalis and patent ductus arteriosus.

b. Ventricular and atrial septal defects and tetralogy of Fallot.

c. Coarctation of the aorta and transposition of the great vessels.

d. All of the above

FILL IN THE BLANK.

11. _____ is a condition caused by an Rh factor or ABO incompatibility.

12. _____ is the failure of one or both testes to descend into the scrotal sac from the abdominal cavity.

13. _____ of the bladder is a congenital malformation in which the lower portion of the abdominal wall and the anterior wall of the bladder are missing.

14. _____ is another term for clubfoot.

15. _____ is the bulging of the ureter into the urinary bladder.

EVALUATE EACH STATEMENT. WRITE A *T* FOR TRUE OR AN *F* FOR FALSE ON THE LINE PROVIDED.

16. ___ Duplicated ureter means that each kidney has two ureters.

17. ___ There are four basic forms of talipes.

18. ___ Hip dysplasia requires early treatment to prevent permanent disability.

24

19. ___ Cystic fibrosis is a congenital disorder of the endocrine glands.

20. ___ PKU is treated by following a carbohydrate-restrictive diet.

Answers

Chapter 4: Congenital Diseases

1. b (p. 57)

2. a (p. 59)

3. d   (p. 61)

4. b (p. 64)

5. d (p. 66)

6. c (p. 57)

7. d (p. 57-58)

8. d (p. 58-59)

9. d (p. 59-60)

10. d (p. 60-64)

11. Erythroblastosis fetalis (p. 60)

12. Cryptorchidism (p. 64)

13. Exstrophy (p. 65)

14. Talipes (p. 65)

15. Ureterocele (p. 65)

16. True (p. 64)

17. True (p. 65)

18. True (p. 66)

19. False (p. 66)

20. False (p. 67)

CHAPTER 5: URINARY SYSTEM DISEASES

Chapter Goal

To inform students of the description, etiology, signs and symptoms, diagnostic procedures, treatment, prognosis, and prevention of the most common diseases of the urinary system.

Learning Objectives

Upon successful completion of the chapter and class lecture and discussion, students will respond to the following on a written exam within the allotted class time with a minimum of _____% accuracy:

- Identify the major diseases of the kidney.
- Name the most common diagnostic procedures used to detect kidney and kidney-related diseases.
- List at least three characteristics common to polycystic kidney disease.
- Identify complications of kidney-related diseases.
- Compare and contrast pyelonephritis and glomerulonephritis.
- Recall infectious precursors to kidney-related diseases.
- Explain why women are more prone to urinary tract infections.
- List the characteristics unique to nephrotic syndrome.
- Name at least three causes of uremia.
- Describe how acute tubular necrosis occurs.
- Discuss the complications of renal calculi.
- Identify possible treatments for renal calculi.
- Repeat the common signs and symptoms of urinary infections.
- Define neurogenic bladder.
- Compare and contrast malignant tumors of the bladder and kidney.
- Distinguish between the two types of kidney dialysis.
- List at least four common urinary system complaints.

Class Activities

Since this is the first chapter of the text that can be easily identified with the specific body system, you will need to make a decision about how to introduce the material in class. It is most easily presented as a module either following or introduced by the terminology and anatomy of the urinary system. In either format, a review of the organs of the urinary system is helpful and necessary. In some class settings, it would even be appropriate to include basic laboratory skills related to the collection of urine for diagnostic purposes.

Name_____

Test Questions

Chapter 5: Urinary System Diseases

CIRCLE THE ONE BEST ANSWER.

1. During a physical examination to diagnosis polycystic kidney disease, the physician may find
a. Atrophied kidneys.
b. Hypertension.
c. Nephritis.
d. Lower than normal body temperature

2. Symptoms of pyelonephritis include all of the following except
a. Pyuria.
b. Dysuria.
c. Nocturia.
d. Glycosuria.

3. Glomerulonephritis usually follows which of the following?
a. AIDS
b. Strep middle ear infection
c. Staph influenza
d. A birth defect

4. Nephrotic syndrome is characterized by severe
a. Proteinuria.
b. Nocturia.
c. Polyuria.
d. Dysuria.

5. Incontinence is the
a. Inability of the kidneys to produce urine.
b. Common symptom of neurogenic bladder.
c. Inability to control urination.
d. b and c

6. The challenge in treating adenocarcinoma of the kidney is that
a. The client typically remains asymptomatic until the later stages of the disease.
b. The client becomes anemic soon after diagnosis.
c. The client is unable to form urine.
d. None of the above .

7. Polycystic kidney failure
a. Causes fluid-filled sacs or cysts in the renal pelvis.

b. Is usually asymptomatic until midlife.
c. a and b
d. None of the above

8. Acute pyelonephritis is
a. Inflammation of the kidney and renal pelvis.
b. Due to infection, most commonly the Escherichia coli bacteria.
c. Determined partly by culture and sensitivity tests on a clean-catch urine specimen.
d. All of the above

9. Common symptoms of urinary diseases include
a. Breathing irregularities and productive cough.
b. Blood in feces.
c. Malaise, fatigue, and lethargy.
d. a and b

10. The allergic inflammation of the glomeruli in the kidney's nephrons is
a. Nephrotic syndrome.
b. Atelectasis.
c. Cholecystitis.
d. Glomerulonephritis.

11. Acute glomerulonephritis
a. May reveal "bloody," "coffee-colored," or "smoky" urine upon diagnostic testing.
b. Usually follows a respiratory streptococcal infection.
c. Reduces the rate of filtration of the blood, causing retention of water and salts.
d. All of the above

FILL IN THE BLANK.

12. Gradual, progressive deterioration of kidney function is called chronic renal failure or
_____.

13. Rapid destruction or degeneration of the tubular segments of nephrons in the kidneys is called ATN or _____.

14. Ultrasonic percutaneous lithotripsy is a treatment for kidney stones that _____. (Describe the action.)

15. _____ is the distension of the renal pelvis and calyces of a kidney due to pressure from accumulating urine.

16. Common lower urinary tract infections (UTIs) are _____ and _____.

17. Any loss or impairment of bladder function caused by central nervous system injury or damage to nerves supplying the bladder is called _____.

18. _____ is a process in which water-soluble substances diffuse across a semipermeable membrane.

EVALUATE EACH STATEMENT. WRITE A *T* FOR TRUE OR AN *F* FOR FALSE ON THE LINE PROVIDED.

19. ___ Tumors of the bladder are almost always malignant.

20. ___ Hemodialysis uses a person's own peritoneum as the dialyzing membrane.

21. ___ Every transplanted kidney contains antigens foreign to the recipient, unless it is donated by an identical twin.

22. ___ Infection by the bacterial Escherichia coli accounts for the majority of UTIs.

23. ___ Hypernephroma seldom metastasizes.

24. ___ Nausea and vomiting or anorexia are not symptoms of urinary system diseases.

Answers

Chapter 5: Urinary System Diseases

1. b (p. 73)

2. d (p. 78)

3. b (p. 79)

4. a (p. 79-80)

5. d (p. 84)

6. a (p. 85)

7. c (p. 73)

8. d (p. 78-79)

9. c (p. 88)

10. d (p. 79)

11. d (p. 79)

12. uremia (p. 80)

13. acute tubular necrosis (p. 81)

14. pulverizes the stones in place, allowing them to be passed in the urine (p. 82)

15. Hydronephrosis (p. 83)

16. cystitis and urethritis (p. 83)

17. neurogenic bladder (p. 84)

18. Dialysis (p. 86)

19. True (p. 85)

20. False (p. 86)

21. True (p. 88)

22. True (p. 83)

23. False (p. 85)

24. False (p. 88)

Answers to the case studies in chapter 5

I. 27-year-old man
1. Diagnostic tests to consider:
a. urine culture and sensitivity
b. microscopic urinalysis
c. complete patient history
2. Effective measures include:
a. maintaining adequate fluid intake
b. emptying the bladder regularly
c. avoiding "holding" urine
d. drinking juices, such as cranberry, to acidify the urine

II. 35-year-old woman
1. Questions to ask:
a. When did this problem begin?
b. How would you describe the pain?
c. Have you been running a fever?
d. How frequently and in what quantities are you urinating?
e. Have you had urinary problems before?
f. Are you on any medications?
2. Diagnostic tests to consider:
a. Refer to Case I diagnostic tests.
3. Preventive measures include:
a. Refer to Case I measures, with the addition of advising the woman to practice proper feminine hygiene.

CHAPTER 6: REPRODUCTIVE SYSTEM DISEASES

Chapter Goal

To inform students of the description, etiology, signs and symptoms, diagnostic procedures, treatment, prognosis, and prevention of the most common diseases of the male and female reproductive systems.

Learning Objectives

Upon successful completion of the chapter and class lecture and discussion, students will respond to the following in a written exam within the allotted class time with a minimum of ____% accuracy:

- Describe the twofold function of human sexuality.
- List the three components of sexual health identified by the World Health Organization.
- Discuss the three factors that cause dyspareunia.
- Compare erectile dysfunction (impotence) in men to arousal and orgasmic dysfunction in women.
- Identify the possible causes for premature ejaculation.
- List the factors that contribute to both female and male fertility.
- Identify the classic symptoms of infertility.
- Discuss diagnostic procedures used to identify infertility in men and women.
- Describe the necessity for a complete sexual history when obtaining a patient's medical history.
- List the seven sexually transmitted diseases (STDs).
- Contrast the causes of STDs.
- Identify the diseases related to the prostate gland.
- Discuss the complications of prostate-related disorders.
- Restate the common causes of epididymitis and orchitis.
- Compare the diseases related to female menses.
- List the characteristic signs and symptoms of ovarian cysts or tumors.
- Define endometriosis.
- Identify a primary complication of endometriosis.
- Describe the most common tumor in women.
- List the causes of pelvic inflammatory disease.
- Discuss the signs and symptoms of menopause.
- Identify the procedures used for diagnosing breast-related diseases.
- List the three reasons for breast reconstruction.
- Recall the possible causes of spontaneous abortion.
- Define ectopic pregnancy.
- Compare preeclampsia with eclampsia.
- Compare placenta previa with abruptio placentae.
- Define PROM.
- List the most common reasons for cesarean birth.
- Recall at least six common reproductive system complaints.

Class Activities

The introduction to this chapter found in the text will help set the tone of class presentations on reproductive system diseases. While students often consider themselves well informed regarding reproductive system diseases, they are more often misinformed.

Sexual dysfunction, infertility, and sexually transmitted diseases may be presented before or after the diseases related specifically to the male and female reproductive systems. An enormous amount of educational material is available on these topics. You may also want to use speakers from public health clinics or Planned Parenthood.

Name_____

Test Questions

Chapter 6: Reproductive System Diseases

CIRCLE THE ONE BEST ANSWER.

1. Physiological factors that can cause arousal and orgasmic dysfunction include
a. Diabetes mellitus.
b. Multiple sclerosis.
c. All of the above
d. None of the above

2. The Huhner test is performed to diagnose
a. Gonorrhea.
b. Infertility.
c. Cervicitis.
d. Papillomas.

3. Which of the following statements regarding infertility is false?
a. It is diagnosed as the failure to become pregnant after 1 year of regular, unprotected intercourse.
b. About 10 percent of couples in the United States are infertile.
c. Fertility peaks for females at 24 years and males at 25 years of age.
d. Men are most fertile when they have intercourse four times a week.

4. Sexually transmitted diseases (STDs) include
a. Genital warts.
b. Trichomoniasis.
c. Chlamydia.
d. All of the above

5. The cause of prostatitis is
a. STDs.
b. Bacteria.
c. Nonbacterial.
d. b and c

6. The prognosis for testicular cancer is
a. 20% cure rate if detected early.
b. 90% cure rate if detected early.
c. 100% cure rate.
d. Grave.

7. An ovarian cyst is derived from
a. Uterine ligaments.

b. Ovarian follicles.

c. The corpus luteum.

d. b and c.

8. The cause of endometriosis is

a. UTIs.

b. Cancer.

c. Ovarian cysts.

d. Unknown.

9. Endometriosis is

a. Caused by fibroid tumors.

b. Infection of the fallopian tubes.

c. Growth of endometrial tissue outside the endometrium.

d. Not accompanied by pain.

10. Symptoms of mammary dysplasia include

a. Lumpiness or a localized mass in the breast.

b. Lower abdominal or pelvic pain.

c. Pain, tenderness, or nipple discharge.

d. a and c.

11. Women at increased risk of breast cancer include

a. Those who remained childless at age 40.

b. Those with a history of chronic breast disease.

c. Those exposed to high radiation doses.

d. All of the above.

12. The most common disorders of pregnancy are

a. Spontaneous abortion and ectopic pregnancy.

b. Benign fibroadenoma and endometriosis.

c. Premature rupture of membranes (PROM) and abruptio placentae.

d. a and c.

13. A blood test that can indicate prostatic cancer is

a. RPR.

b. VDRL.

c. PSA.

d. C and S.

14. Which of the following can be a cause of dyspareunia?

a. Deformities of the vagina

b. Genitourinary tract infections

c. Feelings of guilt or shame

d. All of the above

15. Erectile dysfunction can be caused by

a. Drug and alcohol abuse.

b. Spinal cord injuries.

c. All of the above
d. None of the above

16. A new treatment for erectile dysfunction in men that has about a 70% success rate is
a. Psychotherapy.
b. Viagra.
c. Penile prosthesis.
d. None of the above

17. In men, which condition can be a complication of infection with the mumps virus?
a. Benign prostatic hyperplasia (BPH)
b. Prostatic carcinoma
c. Orchitis
d. Urethritis

18. A predisposing factor for testicular cancer is
a. Increasing age.
b. Cryptorchidism.
c. Hypospadias.
d. BPH

19. Testicular cancer is most common
a. After the age of 40 years.
b. In men with BPH.
c. Before the age of 40 years.
d. In men who have not be circumcised.

20. Premenstrual syndrome (PMS) occurs most frequently in
a. Men after the age of 50 years.
b. Women who have not had children.
c. Women before the age of 20 years.
d. Women in their thirties and forties.

21. The cessation of menses, usually between the ages of 40 and 50 years is
a. Menopause.
b. Menorrhagia.
c. Endometriosis.
d. Menarche.

22. Painful intercourse is
a. Coitus.
b. Impotence.
c. Dyspareunia.
d. Cervicitis.

23. Inability to achieve or sustain penile erection is
a. Impotence.
b. Syphilis.
c. Frigidity.

d. None of the above.

24. One of the most prevalent STDs in the United States is
a. Syphilis.
b. Genital herpes.
c. Genital warts.
d. Gonorrhea.

25. Pregnancy failure after 1 year of regular, unprotected sexual intercourse is referred to as
a. Impotence.
b. Frigidity.
c. Infertility.
d. Dyspareunia.

26. Another term for sexual intercourse is
a. Orgasm.
b. Coitus.
c. Ejaculation.
d. Prostatitis.

27. Which of the following has no cure?
a. Trichomoniasis
b. Genital warts
c. Syphilis
d. Genital herpes

28. A chancre appears in the primary stage of
a. Azoospermia.
b. Syphilis.
c. Genital warts.
d. Gonorrhea.

29. Which may help to prevent the spread of STDs?
a. Condoms
b. Hormone therapy
c. Cryosurgery
d. Chlamydia

30. The function(s) of human sexuality is (are)
a. Enhancement of caring and pleasure.
b. Reproduction.
c. Protection from sexual dysfunction.
d. a and b

31. Considerations in the treatment of any sexual dysfunction include
a. Open communication between client and physician.
b. Conducting a detailed sexual history as part of the medical history.
c. Alertness to signals and questions that may indicate a sexual concern.

38

d. All of the above.

32. Common symptoms of disorders of pregnancy and delivery are
a. Abdominal pain, tenderness, and cramping.
b. Unusual pink or brown discharge or clots.
c. Hypertension, rapid weight gain, edema, and malaise.
d. All of the above

EVALUATE EACH STATEMENT. WRITE A *T* FOR TRUE OR AN *F* FOR FALSE ON THE LINE PROVIDED.

33. ___ Chlamydia infection is sometimes called the "silent" STD.

34. ___ Prostatitis is more common in men younger than 50 years of age.

35. ___ Epididymitis is typically unilateral.

36. ___ Orchitis typically arises as a consequence of rubeola.

37. ___ BPH refers to benign prostaglandin hydrocele.

38. ___ PMS is a cluster of symptoms that recur prior to menstruation.

39. ___ Amenorrhea refers to the absence of menstruation.

40. ___ Metrorrhagia is excessive menstrual flow.

41. ___ Laparoscopy and sonography may be used to diagnose ovarian cysts and tumors.

Answers

Chapter 6: Reproductive System Diseases

1. c (p. 97)

2. b (p. 98)

3. c (p. 98)

4. d (p. 99-104)

5. d (p. 104)

6. b (p. 108)

7. d (p. 111)

8. d (p. 112)

9. c (p. 112)

10. d (p. 115)

11. d (p. 116)

12. d (p. 118-121)

13. c (p. 108)

14. d (p. 96)

15. c (p. 96)

16. b (p. 97)

17. c (p. 107)

18. b (p. 108)

19. c (p. 108)

20. d (p. 109)

21. a (p. 114)

22. c (p. 96)

23. a (p. 96)

24. d (p. 99)

25. c (p. 98)

26. b (p. 99)

27. d (p. 101)

28. b (p. 102)

29. a (p. 103)

30. d (p. 95)

31. d (p. 96)

32. d (p. 122)

33. True (104)

34. False (p. 104)

35. True (p. 105)

36. False (p. 107)

37. False (p. 107)

38. True (p. 109)

39. True (p. 111)

40. False (p. 113)

41. True (p. 112)

Answers to the case studies in chapter 6

I. 15-year-old girl
   1. The young woman should be advised to make an appointment with the physician because her symptoms may be indicative of more than a urinary tract infection (UTI.).
   2. The young woman's symptoms may indicate a UTI or gonorrhea, although vaginal discharge is not a common symptom of UTI.
   3. Diagnostic tests for UTI are microscopic urinalysis and culture and sensitivity tests. The diagnostic test for gonorrhea is a bacteria culture from the site of infection.

II. 51-year-old woman
   1. The woman's age indicates that she may be suffering menopausal symptoms.
   2. The physician would order a test for estrogen/progesterone blood levels and might want to do additional hormonal testing.
   3. Hot flashes may occur during or after menopause as the result of vessel disturbances that accompany hormonal changes in the ovaries, hypothalamus, and pituitary.

III. 38-year-old woman
   1. The recommendation of the American Cancer Society is that the mammogram is one of the best screening devices for the presence of abnormal growths in the breast.
   2. Pain and tenderness can be a symptom of breast cancer.
   3. Offer this woman printed information of signs and symptoms of breast disease and caution her to return immediately should any of these symptoms occur.
      An immediate mammogram and a second opinion are options.

CHAPTER 7: DIGESTIVE SYSTEM DISEASES

Chapter Goal

To inform students of the description, etiology, signs and symptoms, diagnostic procedures, treatment, prognosis, and prevention of the most common diseases of the digestive system.

Learning Objectives

Upon successful completion of the chapter and class lecture and discussion, the student will respond to the following in a written exam within the allotted class time with a minimum of _____% accuracy.

- Define stomatitis.
- List three types of hiatal hernias.
- Identify at least four causes of gastritis.
- Discuss the signs and symptoms of gastroenteritis.
- Describe the destructive process that causes gastric ulcers.
- Describe the steps to be taken for prevention of *E. coli* infections.
- Describe the symptoms of appendicitis.
- Discuss the inflammatory pattern of Crohn's disease.
- List at least three predisposing factors of ulcerative colitis.
- Restate the cause of, and treatment for, abdominal hernias.
- Identify populations at high risk for colorectal cancer.
- Describe the condition of hemorrhoids.
- Compare and contrast anorexia nervosa and bulimia.
- Explain the symptoms of malabsorption syndrome.
- Define duodenal ulcer.
- Discuss the treatment of duodenal ulcers.
- Review causes of irritable bowel syndrome.
- Describe diarrhea as a symptom.
- Explain the implications of pancreatitis.
- Recall the incidence of pancreatic cancer.
- Discuss the relationship between cholecystitis and cholelithiasis.
- Describe cirrhosis and its treatment.
- Name two complications of cirrhosis.
- Define the different types of hepatitis.
- Discuss the etiology of colic.
- Compare and contrast acute and chronic diarrhea.
- List the most common nutritional allergens.
- Compare and contrast roundworm and pinworm infestations.
- List at least three common digestive system complaints.

Class Activities

Diseases of the digestive system are common, significant, and varied in characteristics. You will be able to find a great deal of additional material on any of the diseases presented here if you choose to use it.

You may want to separate the class presentations into upper gastrointestinal (GI) tract diseases, lower GI tract diseases, diseases of accessory organs of digestion, and childhood diseases related to the digestive system. If speakers are available to you, consider asking a physician of internal medicine or a gastroenterologist to speak to your class.

NAME_____

Test Questions

Chapter 7: Digestive System Diseases

CIRCLE THE ONE BEST ANSWER.

1. Acute stomatitis is caused by
a. Herpes simplex type 2.
b. Herpes simplex type 1.
c. Genital herpes.
d. Bacterial infections.

2. Gastritis is confirmed by
a. Gastroscopy with biopsy.
b. Blood tests.
c. Urine tests.
d. Blood smear.

3. Traveler's diarrhea is also known as
a. Gastric ulcer.
b. Gastritis.
c. Gastroenteritis.
d. Enteritis.

4. Contributing factors to a gastric ulcer include
a. Smoking.
b. Salicylate reaction.
c. Increased stress.
d. All of the above

5. Signs and symptoms of a hiatal hernia include
a. Gastritis.
b. Heartburn.
c. Diarrhea.
d. Vomiting.

6. Treatment of celiac sprue is a
a. Glucose-free diet.
b. Low calorie diet.
c. Fat free diet.
d. Gluten-free diet.

7. The most frequently occurring gastrointestinal (GI) disorder is
a. Diverticulitis.
b. Irritable bowel syndrome.

c. Duodenal ulcer.

d. Hiatal hernia.

8. Crohn's disease most often affects the

a. Cecum.

b. Transverse colon.

c. Jejunum.

d. Ileum.

9. The definitive method of diagnosing Crohn's disease is through

a. Colonoscopy.

b. Biopsy of the affected site.

c. Ileostomy.

d. Barium enema.

10. The leading cause of chronic pancreatitis is

a. Acute pancreatitis.

b. Gallstones.

c. Alcoholism.

d. Chronic diverticulitis.

11. Proponents of alternative medicine identify the following factors to consider in digestive disorders

a. Food allergies, psychological stress, insufficient exercise, and a compromised immune system

b. Food allergies and insufficient exercise only.

c. Insufficient exercise and psychological stress only.

d. None of the above

12. Gastritis

a. In its acute form may cause belching, gastrointestinal bleeding, epigastric pain, and hematemesis or vomiting.

b. Has a good prognosis with proper treatment.

c. May require gastroscopy and x-ray for diagnosis.

d. All of the above

13. Peptic ulcers

a. Are found in the stomach and duodenum.

b. Are the result of gluten-induced enteropathy.

c. Are treated by the avoidance of alcohol, caffeine, and smoking.

d. a and c

14. Hernias

a. Are life-threatening.

b. Are usually the result of weakness in the musculature.

c. May strangulate without proper treatment.

d. b and c

15. Celiac sprue

a. Is a disease of the colon.

b. Is easy to diagnose because of severe pain in the stomach.

c. Affects men twice as frequently as women.

d. Is treated with a gluten-free diet.

16. Aphthous stomatitis is

a. Caused by herpes simplex 1.

b. Caused by unknown factors.

c. Unlikely to cause difficulty chewing, swallowing, or speaking.

d. Usually related to an STD.

17. Fecal occult blood testing is performed to screen for

a. Gastric ulcer.

b. Aphthous stomatitis.

c. Colorectal cancer.

d. Cirrhosis.

18. The fifth leading cause of cancer deaths, which produces symptoms of abdominal pain, anorexia, weight loss, and blood glucose abnormalities, usually in people over 60 years of age, is

a. Cirrhosis.

b. Pancreatic cancer.

c. Colorectal cancer.

d. Cholelithiasis.

19. Dilated, tortuous veins in anal or rectal mucous membranes are

a. Irritable bowel syndrome.

b. Hemorrhoids.

c. Diverticulitis.

d. Cholelithiasis.

20. The most frequently occurring gastrointestinal disorder in United States is

a. Ulcerative colitis.

b. Acute pancreatitis.

c. Irritable bowel syndrome.

d. Abdominal hernia.

21. Tenderness on pressure at McBurney's point is a diagnostic indicator of

a. Acute pancreatitis.

b. Cirrhosis

c. Diverticulitis.

d. Acute appendicitis.

22. Bloody diarrhea, often containing pus and mucus, is a classic symptom of

a. Pruritus.

b. Ulcerative colitis

c. Colorectal cancer.

d. None of the above.

23. Inflammation through all layers of the intestinal wall resulting in thickening of the wall and narrowing of the lumen is
a. Crohn's disease.
b. Diverticulitis.
c. Acute cholecystitis.
d. Aphthous stomatitis.

24. An autodigestive process that is severe, often life threatening, is
a. Pancreatic cancer.
b. Ulcerative colitis.
c. Acute pancreatitis.
d. Duodenal ulcer.

25. Acute inflammation of small, pouchlike herniations in the intestinal wall is
a. Cirrhosis.
b. Crohn's disease.
c. Duodenal ulcer.
d. Diverticulitis.

26. Slow, progressive destruction of pancreatic tissue is
a. Acute pancreatitis.
b. Chronic pancreatitis.
c. Diverticulitis.
d. Pancreatic cancer.

27. The diagnostic procedure(s) most likely used to diagnose colorectal cancer is (are)
a. Digital examination of the rectum and barium x-ray.
b. Testing for occult blood in the stool and sigmoidoscopy.
c. Colonoscopy.
d. All of the above

28. Possible complications of diarrhea are
a. Dehydration.
b. Electrolyte imbalances.
c. Dysuria.
d. a and b

FILL IN THE BLANK.

29. _____ is apt to cause three times more deaths in the next decade.

30. _____ is paroxysmal abdominal pain or cramping occurring during the first few months of life.

31. _____ are common childhood food allergens.

32. Methods of preventing worm infestations include _____ and _____.

EVALUATE EACH STATEMENT. WRITE A *T* FOR TRUE OR AN *F* FOR FALSE ON THE LINE PROVIDED.

33. ___ Pancreatic cancer usually occurs in the tail of the pancreas.

34. ___ Cholelithiasis refers to gallstones in the gallbladder or bile ducts.

35. ___ The treatment of choice for acute cholecystitis is cholecystectomy.

36. ___ A chronic, reversible disease of the liver is called cirrhosis.

37. ___ Hepatitis A virus is a common threat to health-care workers.

38. ___ There is no one specific treatment for hepatitis.

39. ___ An eating disorder characterized by an all-consuming desire to remain thin is called bulimia.

40. ___ Bulimic persons typically have a high incidence of dental caries.

41. ___ Common symptoms of digestive system diseases are loss of appetite, weight loss, nausea, and vomiting.

42. ___ Men are rarely afflicted with anorexia nervosa.

48

Answers

Chapter 7: Digestive System Diseases

1. b (p. 129)

2. a (p. 129)

3. c (p. 131)

4. d (p. 131-132)

5. b (p. 133)

6. d (p. 134)

7. b (p. 136)

8. d (p. 137)

9. b (p. 137)

10. c (p. 144)

11. a (p. 152)

12. d (p. 129)

13. d (p. 131-132)

14. d (p. 132-133)

15. d (p. 134)

16. b (p. 129)

17. c (p. 141)

18. b (p. 144)

19. b (p. 139)

20. c (p. 136)

21. d (p. 136)

22. b (p. 138)

23. a (p. 137)

24. c (p. 142)

25. d (p. 138)

26. b (p. 143)

27. d (p. 141)

28. d (p. 142)

29. Hepatitis C (p. 148)

30. Infantile colic (p. 150)

31. Milk products, eggs, and wheat (p. 151)

32. handwashing, keeping fungi out of the mouth (p. 152)

33. False (p. 144)

34. True (p. 144)

35. True (p. 146)

36. False (p. 147)

37. False (p. 149)

38. True (p. 148)

39. False (p. 149)

40. True (p. 150)

41. True (p. 152)

42. True (p. 149)

Answers to the case studies in chapter 7

I. 52-year-old man
   1. Irritable bowel syndrome (IBS) is a chronic digestive tract disease marked by abdominal pain and altered bowel function.

2. The reported symptoms are not characteristic of IBS. The hallmark indication of IBS is abdominal pain with constipation or constipation alternating with diarrhea.
3. The most significant symptom is the bloody diarrhea.
4. The tests most likely to be ordered are sigmoidoscopy, colonoscopy, barium enema, and rectal biopsy.

II. 35-year-old woman
  1. The physician is apt to do a complete physical examination, which might include a small intestine biopsy and blood tests to determine any mineral and/or vitamin deficiencies.

CHAPTER 8: RESPIRATORY SYSTEM DISEASES

Chapter Goal

To inform students of the description, etiology, signs and symptoms, diagnostic procedures, treatment, prognosis, and prevention of the most common diseases of the respiratory system.

Learning Objectives

Upon successful completion of the chapter and class lecture and discussion, the student will respond to the following on a written exam within the allotted class time with a minimum of _____% accuracy.

- Define epistaxis.
- List the causes of sinusitis.
- Describe the treatment for laryngitis.
- Identify the confirming diagnosis of mononucleosis.
- Contrast the three types of pneumonia.
- Describe the conditions under which a lung abscess may occur.
- Explain the treatment modalities for pneumothorax.
- Define pleurisy.
- Differentiate between transudate and exudate fluid.
- Name the most common chronic lung disease.
- List the predisposing factors of chronic bronchitis.
- Recall the signs and symptoms of emphysema.
- Discuss the prognosis for asthma.
- Explain the growth of the tuberculosis bacteria.
- Compare the four pneumoconioses.
- Review the etiology of SIDS.
- Report the treatment of choice for chronic tonsillitis and adenoid hyperplasia.
- Describe the signs and symptoms of croup.
- Identify the etiology of acute epiglottitis.

Class Activities

Regardless of the specialty or general practice in which they work, allied health professionals see many respiratory diseases in their professional careers and therefore need adequate training in this area. Keep in mind that it is helpful to review the anatomy and physiology of a particular system before beginning a serious discussion of its pathophysiology.

As with other systems, it is helpful to access other resources to use in your class. Check for suggestions of relevant audiovisual materials and seek the assistance of outside speakers if you wish. Those especially helpful in this area include internal medicine physicians who specialize in pulmonary diseases, respiratory therapists, or any patient who suffers from a chronic lung disease.

Name_____

Test Questions

Chapter 8: Respiratory System Diseases

SELECT THE ONE BEST ANSWER:

1. Infectious mononucleosis is caused by
a. Human immunodeficiency virus (HIV).
b. Hemophilus influenzae.
c. Epstein Barr virus.
d. Bacteria.

2. Initial symptoms of mononucleosis include
a. Sore throat.
b. Malaise and chills.
c. Swollen cervical lymph nodes.
d. All of the above

3. Pneumonia is caused by
a. Viruses or bacteria.
b. Protozoa or rickettsiae.
c. a and b
d. None of the above

4. Pneumonia affects
a. Trachea.
b. Bronchioles.
c. Alveolar ducts.
d. b and c

5. A complication of influenza-caused pneumonia is
a. Pneumothorax.
b. Asthma.
c. Bronchitis.
d. Lung abscess.

6. Lung abscesses are normally found in the
a. Right lower lobe.
b. Left lower lobe.
c. Right upper lobe.
d. Left upper lobe

7. A collection of air in the pleural cavity is
a. Pleurisy.
b. Pleural effusion.

c. Pneumothorax.

d. Chronic obstructive pulmonary disease (COPD).

8. Symptoms of pleurisy include

a. Purulent sputum.

b. Collapsed lung.

c. Bleeding.

d. Sharp, stabbing chest pain.

9. For bronchitis to be diagnosed as chronic, a productive cough must be

a. Present for 3 months of the year over at least 2 consecutive years.

b. Present for 1 year without responding to treatment.

c. Present for two years along with edema and cyanosis.

d. Treated for 6 months without a cure

10. Emergency treatment for asthma includes

a. Oxygen.

b. Bronchodilators.

c. Antihistamines.

d. a and b

11. Pulmonary tuberculosis is more common in

a. Children.

b. Young adults.

c. Middle-aged adults.

d. Elderly adults.

12. Persons who have a positive tuberculin reaction

a. Are treated with antibiotics.

b. Are tested for pulmonary tuberculosis (TB) after 2 months.

c. Are given a year of isoniazid prophylactically.

d. None of the above

13. Diseases that are classified as Pneumoconiosis include

a. Berylliosis.

b. Histoplasmosis.

c. Mycoses.

d. b and c

14. Anthracosis is caused by

a. Bird and chicken droppings.

b. Inhaling asbestos fibers.

c. Inhaling coal dust.

d. Inhaling fungal spores in the desert.

15. Cor pulmonale

a. Is fatal.

b. Can not be prevented.

c. Can be chronic.

54

d. b and c

16. Radiation exposure can result in
a. Bronchiectasis.
b. Lung cancer.
c. Cor pulmonale.
d. Anthracosis.

17. The antibiotic of choice for acute tonsillitis is
a. Erythromycin.
b. EES.
c. Keflex.
d. Penicillin.

18. Excessive alkalinity of body fluids caused by excessive removal of carbon dioxide by the lungs is known as
a. Respiratory acidosis.
b. Respiratory alkalosis.
c. Atelectasis.
d. Cor pulmonale.

19. Sudden Infant Death Syndrome (SIDS) occurs
a. In apparently normal and healthy infants.
b. More frequently when the infant is sleeping and in premature infants.
c. More frequently in male than in female infants and during the winter months.
d. All of the above

20. Cor pulmonale is
a. A mass of undissolved matter in the pulmonary artery.
b. A form of pneumonoconiosis.
c. An accumulation of fluid in the pulmonary tissues.
d. Hypertrophy and failure of the right ventricle of the heart.

21. Respiratory mycoses affecting the lungs are
a. Histoplasmosis, coccidioidomycosis, and blastomycosis.
b. Pneumonoconiosis, blastomycosis, and histoplasmosis.
c. Anthracosis, coccidioidomycosis, and pneumonoconiosis.
d. Anthracosis, berylliosis, and asbestosis.

22. Lung cancer
a. Is the leading cause of cancer deaths in women over 40.
b. Causes dyspnea and hemoptysis in the early stages.
c. Has a poor prognosis.
d. a and c

23. A pulmonary embolism
a. Generally originates in the pelvic or deep lower-extremity veins.
b. Travels through the circulatory system until it blocks an artery.
c. Causes pneumonia-like symptoms.

d. b and c

24. Which of the following childhood diseases may require emergency tracheostomy or endotracheal intubation?
a. Croup
b. Acute epiglottitis
c. Acute tonsillitis
d. Adenoid hyperplasia

25. Which of the following statements about tonsillitis is not true?
a. Tonsillitis is an inflammation of the tonsils, especially the palatine tonsils.
b. Most infections are caused by members of the Orthomyxoviridae family.
c. The onset is generally slow and is marked by symptoms of chills and fever.
d. b and c

26. Common symptoms of croup include
a. Hoarseness, fever, and distinctive hard cough.
b. Persistent stridor and respiratory distress.
c. Sore throat and headache.
d. a and b

27. An acute infection of the lung and the sixth leading cause of death in the United States is
a. Asthma.
b. COPD.
c. Pneumothorax.
d. Pneumonia.

28. Inflammation of the parietal and visceral pleurae is
a. Pleurisy.
b. Asthma.
c. COPD.
d. Bronchitis.

29. Intrinsic asthma
a. Is most common in children.
b. Is caused by allergies.
c. Is caused by psychosomatic disorders.
d. Is most common in adults.

30. Acute or chronic hyperventilation can cause
a. Respiratory acidosis.
b. Asthma.
c. Respiratory alkalosis.
d. Cor pulmonale.

31. Inflammation of the pharynx is
a. Stenosis.
b. Pharyngitis.

c. Laryngitis.
d. None of the above.

32. Inflammation of the respiratory bronchioles, alveolar ducts, alveolar sacs, and alveoli of the lungs is
a. Pulmonary TB.
b. Pleurisy.
c. Asthma.
d. Pneumonia.

33. A slowly developing bacterial lung infection characterized by progressive necrosis of lung tissue is
a. Pleurisy.
b. Pulmonary TB.
c. COPD.
d. Chronic pulmonary emphysema.

34. Inflammation of the paranasal sinus is
a. Bronchiectasis.
b. Sinusitis.
c. Acute pharyngitis.
d. Epistaxis.

35. Inflammation the visceral and parietal pleural membranes that envelop each lung is
a. Pleural effusion.
b. COPD.
c. Pleurisy.
d. Pneumothorax.

36. Any pathological process that decreases the ability of the lungs and bronchi to perform their function of ventilation is
a. Chronic bronchitis.
b. Bronchiectasis.
c. Chronic obstructive pulmonary disease.
d. Asthma.

37. A form of pneumoconiosis resulting from the inhalation of quartz dust is
a. Pleurisy.
b. Atelectasis.
c. Asbestosis.
d. Silicosis.

38. Permanent abnormal dilation of small and medium-sized bronchi is
a. Respiratory alkalosis.
b. Chronic bronchitis.
c. Bronchiectasis.
d. Atelectasis.

39. Inflammation of the vocal cords and the surrounding bone is
a. Laryngitis.
b. Pharyngitis.
c. Infectious mononucleosis.
d. None of the above

40. Excess of fluid between parietal and visceral pleural membranes is
a. Pneumonia.
b. Pleural effusion.
c. Pleurisy.
d. Pulmonary TB.

41. A respiratory condition marked by recurrent attacks of labored breathing
accompanied by wheezing is
a. Chronic pulmonary emphysema.
b. Respiratory acidosis.
c. Asthma.
d. Chronic bronchitis.

42. The collapse or airless condition of all or part of a lung is
a. Atelectasis.
b. Pulmonary embolism.
c. Pulmonary edema.
d. Bronchiectasis.

EVALUATE EACH STATEMENT. WRITE A *T* FOR TRUE OR AN *F* FOR FALSE ON THE LINE PROVIDED.

43. ___ Those at risk of asbestosis include workers in the specialty metals, semiconductor
and, ceramics industries.

44. ___ Pulmonary edema is not a medical emergency.
Answer: False

45. ___ Bronchiectasis is a reversible condition.

46. ___ A chronic cough and a characteristic "barrel chest" are likely signs of chronic
pulmonary emphysema.

47. ___ Lung abscesses are more frequent in lower portions of the lungs.

DEFINE

49. Hemoptysis:

58

50. Epistaxis:

51. Rales:

52. Thoracentesis:

53. Dyspnea:

Answers

Chapter 8: Respiratory System Diseases

1. c (p. 161)

2. d (p. 161)

3. c (p. 162)

4. d (p. 162)

5. d (p. 162)

6. a (p. 164)

7. c (p. 165)

8. d (p. 166)

9. a (p. 167)

10. d (p. 169)

11. d (p. 169)

12. c (p. 170)

13. a (p. 171)

14. c (p. 172)

15. d (p. 173)

16. b (p. 176)

17. d (p. 178)

18. b (p. 175)

19. d (p. 177)

20. d (p. 173)

21. a (p. 172)

22. d (p. 176)

23. a (p. 174)

24. b (p. 179)

25. d (p. 177)

26. d (p. 178)

27. d (p. 162)

28. a (p. 166)

29. d (p. 169)

30. c (p. 175)

31. b (p. 160)

32. d (p. 162)

33. b (p. 169)

34. b (p. 160)

35. c (p. 166)

36. c (p. 167)

37. d (p. 171)

38. c (p. 176)

39. a (p. 161)

40. b (p. 166)

41. c (p. 168-169)

42. a (p. 175)

43. False (p. 171)

44. False (p. 173)

45. False (p. 176)

46. True (p. 168)

47. True (p. 164)

48. coughing and spitting up blood due to bleeding in the respiratory tract (Glossary)

49. nosebleed (Glossary)

50. abnormal respiratory sound heard on auscultation of lungs produced by the movement of air through secretion-filled or constricted bronchial passages (Glossary)

51. surgical puncture of the chest wall to remove fluid from either of the pleural cavities (Glossary)

52. labored or difficult breathing, generally indicating an insufficient amount of oxygen in the blood (Glossary)

Answers to the case studies in chapter 8

I. 55-year-old man
   1. Predisposing factors and causes:
      a. a long history of cigarette smoking (primary and secondary)
      b. exposure to asbestos fibers for 6 years (primary and secondary)
   2. The patient's symptoms are:
      a. a slightly irritating cough
      b. dyspnea, even at rest
   3. Preventive measures to avoid affecting the health of the spouse include:
      a. workers showering and changing clothes prior to leaving work if the company is responsible for laundering
      b. taking necessary precautions (e.g., wearing a mask, not shaking clothes) if clothes are washed at home
   4. Smoking for such a long time is indicative of chronic respiratory problems that compromise the respiratory system. The additional exposure to asbestos further irritated damaged tissues and membranes.

II. 72-year-old man
   1. The history and symptoms could indicate a neoplasm.
   2. The aspiration of peanut husks, the long history of smoking (primary and secondary), shortness of breath, dyspnea, and a chronic productive, painful cough all point to a possible neoplasm.
   3. The normal aging process makes his lungs more susceptible to pollutants and disease.

CHAPTER 9: CIRCULATORY SYSTEM DISEASES

Chapter Goal

To inform students of the description, etiology, signs and symptoms, diagnostic procedures, treatment, prognosis, and prevention of the most common diseases of the circulatory system.

Learning Objectives

Upon successful completion of the chapter and class lecture and discussion, students will respond to the following on a written exam in the allotted class time with a minimum of _____% accuracy.

- Describe the infectious heart diseases.
- Identify the valvular heart diseases.
- Identify individuals at high risk of developing hypertension.
- Recall the safe time duration of angina pectoris.
- List the classic signs and symptoms of myocardial infarction.
- Describe congestive heart failure.
- List the causes of heart murmur.
- Contrast atherosclerosis to arteriosclerosis.
- Discuss the prevention of thrombophlebitis.
- Describe varicose veins.
- Recall the classic treatment protocol for polycythemia vera.
- Compare seven anemias.
- Discuss the various treatments of leukemia.
- Define lymphedema.
- Compare lymphosarcoma to Hodgkin's disease.
- Define Reye's syndrome.
- List at least four common symptoms of cardiovascular disease.

Class Activities

The diseases of the circulatory system include those involving the blood, the heart, and the lymphatic system. You may choose to teach the chapter according to these arbitrary divisions or some other manner of dividing the material.

Speakers who can offer assistance include cardiologists, cardiac or vascular surgeons, internal medicine physicians who specialize in diseases of the circulatory system EKG technicians, or exercise physiologists. Dieticians can discuss the importance of low-cholesterol, low-fat, and low-salt diets, all of which are important for individuals at risk for certain circulatory diseases. Many communities also have programs to support persons recovering from a myocardial infarction. These programs can provide helpful information to students on the benefits of exercise and stress reduction.

Illustrations, diagrams, and pictures will help students learn the material of this sometimes-confusing system. A model of the heart, especially one that comes apart, can be another useful tool.

Name_____

Test Questions

Chapter 9: Circulatory System Diseases

CIRCLE THE ONE BEST ANSWER.

1. Rheumatic fever is normally found in
a. Children 2 to 4 years of age.
b. Children and adolescents 5 to 15 years of age.
c. Young adults 18 to 20 years of age.
d. Adults 20 to 30 years of age.

2. Chorea is sometimes found in
a. Endocarditis.
b. Myocarditis.
c. Rheumatic fever.
d. Strep throat.

3. Tests used to diagnose rheumatic fever include
a. Antistreptolysin O (ASO).
b. White blood cell count (WBC).
c. Erythrocyte sedimentation rate (ESR).
d. All of the above

4. Rheumatic fever tends to
a. Have an excellent prognosis.
b. Be recurrent within 5 years.
c. Be recurrent within 15 years.
d. Be fatal.

5. The cause of myocarditis can be
a. A side effect of surgery.
b. Smoking.
c. Chronic alcoholism.
d. Arrhythmias.

6. The best method of diagnosing myocarditis is
a. ECG.
b. Echocardiogram.
c. Stress ECG.
d. Biopsy.

7. Mitral valve insufficiency causes
a. Blood to backflow into the left atrium.
b. Blood to backflow into the right atrium.

64

c. Blood to backflow into the aorta.
d. Blood to backflow into the left ventricle.

8. The major difference in symptoms between angina pectoris and myocardial infarction is
a. Length of time the pain continues.
b. Location of pain.
c. Description of pain.
d. b and c

9. Three common types of aneurysms are
a. Abdominal, thoracic, and aortic.
b. Abdominal, aortic, and peripheral.
c. Abdominal, thoracic, and peripheral.
d. Thoracic, pulmonary, and peripheral

10. Intermittent claudication is
a. Limping or lameness.
b. Changes in skin temperature.
c. A shivering sensation.
d. Loss of sensation in the skin.

11. Thrombophlebitis is caused by
a. Infection.
b. Trauma.
c. Prolonged immobility.
d. a and b

12. Megaloblasts are found in
a. Iron deficiency anemia.
b. Pernicious anemia.
c. Folic acid deficiency anemia.
d. Aplastic anemia.

13. Diagnostic procedures for aplastic anemia include
a. Red blood cell count.
b. White blood cell count.
c. Bone marrow studies.
d. All of the above

14. Treatment of pernicious anemia includes
a. Injections of folic acid.
b. Bone marrow transplant.
c. Injections of Vitamin B_{12}.
d. High doses of Vitamin B.

15. Prognosis for acute myeloblastic leukemia is
a. Excellent.
b. Good, with remission lasting many years.

c. Fatal within one to two months after symptoms begin.
d. Usually fatal after one year of diagnosis.

16. A systemic inflammatory disease affecting the joints, heart, central nervous system, and skin is called
a. Valvular heart disease.
b. Rheumatic fever.
c. Lymphedema.
d. Chronic myelocytic leukemia.

17. The following signs or symptoms occur in rheumatic fever
a. Fever, polyarthritis, chorea, and carditis.
b. Fever and carditis only.
c. Polyarthritis and chorea only.
d. Fever and polyarthritis only.

18. An acute or chronic inflammation of the saclike membrane that surrounds the heart is called
a. Pericarditis.
b. Endocarditis.
c. Myocarditis.
d. Neuritis.

19. The classic symptom of pericarditis is
a. Dyspnea.
b. Heart palpitations.
c. Fever.
d. Pleuritic pain.

20. Myocarditis is caused by
a. Bacteria, viruses, and rheumatic fever.
b. Chronic alcoholism.
c. None of the above.
d. All of the above

21. An inflammation of the membrane lining the heart valves characterized by the formation of vegetations is called
a. pericarditis.
b. myocarditis.
c. endocarditis.
d. mitral insufficiency.

22. Heart murmurs may be caused by
a. Blood leaking back through an incompetent valve.
b. Blood forcing its way through a narrowed valve.
c. A rapid diastolic flow.
d. Hemorrhage of blood through the cardiac sphincter.

23. Hypertension may include the following signs and symptoms
a. Dyspnea, angina, weight loss, light-headedness, and weakness.
b. Angina and weight loss only.
c. Light-headedness and weakness only.
d. Light-headedness only.

24. The leading cause of coronary artery disease is
a. Old age.
b. Atherosclerosis.
c. Obesity.
d. Diabetes mellitus.

25. Chest pain resulting from ischemia to a part of the myocardium is called
a. Coronary artery disease.
b. Myocardial infarction.
c. Angina pectoris.
d. Transient ischemic attacks.

26. A life-threatening condition caused by occlusion of coronary arteries with subsequent necrosis of heart muscle is called
a. Coronary artery disease.
b. Angina pectoris.
c. Myocardial infarction.
d. Congestive heart failure.

27. The classic symptom of myocardial infarction is
a. Dyspnea.
b. Crushing chest pain radiating down the arm.
c. Diastolic pressure greater than 90 mmHg.
d. Systolic pressure greater than 180 mmHg.

28. Complications of myocardial infarction include
a. Arrhythmias and congestive heart failure.
b. Cardiogenic shock and mitral regurgitation.
c. Ventricular aneurysm.
d. All of the above

29. Congestive heart failure can result in which of the following?
a. Lymphedema, peripheral edema, and arterial edema only
b. Lymphedema, peripheral edema, arterial edema, and pulmonary edema
c. Peripheral edema and pulmonary edema only
d. Arterial edema only

30. Treatment of congestive heart failure includes
a. Bed rest, diuretics, and vasodilators only.
b. Bed rest and vasodilators only.
c. Diuretics and digitalis only.
d. Bed rest, diuretics, vasodilators, digitalis, and restricted sodium intake.

31. A local dilation of an artery or chamber of the heart due to weakening of its walls is called
a. Myocardial infarction.
b. Aneurysm.
c. Arteriosclerosis.
d. Atherosclerosis.

32. The condition characterized by accumulation of yellowish plaques of cholesterol, lipids,and cellular debris in the inner layers of large- and medium-sized arteries is called
a. Atherosclerosis.
b. Arteriosclerosis.
c. Coronary artery disease.
d. Myocardial infarction.

33. Signs and symptoms of arteriosclerosis include
a. Intermittent claudication.
b. Changes in skin temperature.
c. Bruits over involved arteries.
d. All of the above

34. Inflammation of a vein in conjunction with the formation of a clot is
a. Coronary artery disease.
b. Myocardial infarction.
c. Thrombophlebitis.
d. Varicose veins.

35. Treatment of thrombophlebitis includes
a. Bed rest and vein ligation
b. Elevation of the affected limb.
c. Application of heat over the affected area and elastic wrap on the affected limb.
d. All of the above

36. Varicose veins occur most commonly in the
a. Large veins in the arms.
b. Greater and lesser saphenous veins.
c. Small veins in the upper thighs.
d. Small arterioles of the lower legs.

37. Which of the following is characterized by inadequate reserves of iron in the body and formation of hemoglobin-poor red blood cells?
a. Folic acid deficiency anemia
b. Pernicious anemia
c. Iron deficiency anemia
d. Sickle-cell anemia

38. Which of the following includes etiologic factors of iron deficiency anemia?
a. Menorrhagia and gastrointestinal bleeding only
b. Menorrhagia, gastrointestinal bleeding, excessive blood donation, poor diet, and pregnancy
c. Excessive blood donation and poor diet only

d. None of the above

39. A type of anemia characterized by the appearance of large-sized, abnormal red blood cells as a result of inadequate levels of vitamin B12 is called
a. Folic acid deficiency anemia.
b. Pernicious anemia.
c. Sickle cell anemia.
d. Iron deficiency anemia.

40. A neoplasm characterized by the hyperproliferation of abnormal, immature white cell precursors called blasts is known as
a. Sick-cell anemia.
b. Acute leukemia.
c. Chronic myelocytic leukemia.
d. Lymphedema.

41. An abnormal accumulation of lymph usually in the extremities is called
a. Sickle-cell anemia.
b. Hodgkin's disease.
c. Chronic myelocytic leukemia.
d. Lymphedema.

42. Signs and symptoms of lymphedema include
a. An affected limb that is swollen and hypertrophied.
b. An affected skin that is thickened and fibrotic.
c. An affected limb that is painful and reddened.
d. a and b

43. A neoplastic malignancy of the lymphatic system characterized by painless enlargement of the lymph nodes and spleen is called
a. Lymphosarcoma.
b. Hodgkin's disease.
c. Lymphedema.
d. Chronic leukemia.

44. Rheumatic heart disease usually occurs after
a. Myocardial infarction
b. Streptococcal infection
c. COPD
d. Angioplasty

45. A life-threatening inflammation of the sac surrounding the heart characterized by dyspnea, tachycardia, orthopnea, pallor is
a. Pericarditis.
b. Myocardial infarction.
c. Rheumatic heart disease.
d. Hypertension.

46. Essential hypertension is
a. Considered to be idiopathic.
b. Considered to be an iatrogenic condition.
c. Not associated with lifestyle risk factors.
d. Is not familial.

47. Persistently elevated blood pressure without apparent cause is
a. Secondary hypertension.
b. Cor pulmonale.
c. Essential hypertension.
d. Atherosclerosis.

48. Mortality from myocardial infarction is highest
a. Within the first hour.
b. After angioplasty.
c. After 48 hours.
d. When treatment is started immediately.

49. In women, fatigue, nausea, vomiting, and shortness of breath could indicate
a. Hypertension.
b. Atherosclerosis.
c. Myocardial infarction.
d. Congestive heart failure.

50. Removal of a large section of the myocardium is being done in Brazil, and now in the United States, as
a. A new, controversial treatment for the cardiomegaly associated with congestive heart failure.
b. A treatment for cardiac cancers.
c. An alternative to heart transplant for viral cardiomyopathy.
d. A treatment for essential hypertension.

51. A condition usually caused by exposure to toxins, radiation, or viruses in which the bone marrow stops producing blood cells, resulting in bleeding tendencies and the inability to fight infections, is
a. Sickle cell anemia.
b. Aplastic anemia.
c. Iron deficiency anemia.
d. Thalassemia.

FILL IN THE BLANK.

52. A childhood disease that develops in five stages, beginning with lethargy and vomiting and ending with seizures, flaccidity, and respiratory arrest is called _____.

53. _____ is a chronic blood disorder characterized by an increased number of red blood cells, leukocytosis, thrombocytosis, and increased hemoglobin concentration.

EVALUATE EACH STATEMENT. WRITE A *T* FOR TRUE OR AN *F* FOR FALSE ON THE LINE PROVIDED.

54. ___ Treatment of rheumatic fever is symptomatic and supportive.

55. ___ Rheumatic heart fever cannot be prevented.

56. ___ Endocarditis is most frequently caused by infection from streptococcal bacteria.

57. ___ Endocarditis is curable when treated early with antibiotics.

58. ___ Diseased heart valves may be too large to close completely or too narrow, impeding the flow of blood.

59. ___ Signs and symptoms of mitral insufficiency or stenosis include fever and pleuritis pain.

60. ___ Cardiac catheterization is too risky to attempt for diagnosis of tricuspid insufficiency or stenosis.

61. ___ For stenosis or insufficiency of any of the heart valves, dyspnea and fatigue are common symptoms.

62. ___ The classic signs of an angina attack are burning, squeezing, and tightness of the chest.

63. ___ Nitroglycerin preparations are used for treatment of mitral insufficiency or stenosis.

64. ___ The prognosis for angina pectoris is good.

65. ___ Cardiac arrest is a medical emergency.

66. ___ Treatment of an aneurysm depends on the size and site of the affected artery, the size of the aneurysm, and the likelihood of its rupturing.

67. ___ The prognosis is excellent for aneurysms.

68. ___ Aplastic anemia is a hereditary, chronic type in which abnormal crescent-shaped red blood cells are present.

69. ___ Leukemias are progressive, malignant diseases of the blood-forming organs.

70. ___ Chronic lymphocytic leukemia is characterized by proliferation of abnormal white cell precursors called granulocytes in the bone marrow.

71. ___ Lymphosarcoma is a non-Hodgkin's lymphosarcoma.

Answers

Chapter 9: Circulatory System Diseases

1. b (p. 185)

2. c (p. 187)

3. d (p. 187)

4. b (p. 187)

5. c (p. 188)

6. a (p. 188)

7. a (p. 190)

8. a (p. 195)

9. c (p. 199)

10. a (p. 200)

11. d (p. 201)

12. c (p. 204)

13. d (p. 205)

14. c (p. 205)

15. d (p. 208)

16. b (185)

17. a (p. 187)

18. a (p. 187)

19. d (p. 188)

20. d (p. 188)

21. c (p. 189)

22. d (p. 190)

23. a (p. 193)

24. b (p. 194)

25. c (p. 195)

26. c (p. 195)

27. b (p. 196)

28. d (p. 196)

29. b (p. 197)

30. d (p. 198)

31. b (p. 199)

32. a (p. 200)

33. d (p. 200)

34. c (p. 201)

35. d (p. 201)

36. b (p. 202)

37. c (p. 203)

38. b (p. 203-204)

39. b (p. 205)

40. b (p. 207-208)

41. d (p. 209)

42. d (p. 209-210)

43. b (p. 211)

44. b (p. 185)

45. a (p. 188)

46. a (p. 193)

47. c (p. 193)

48. a (p. 196)

49. d (p. 196)

50. a (p. 198)

51. b (p. 205)

52. Reye's syndrome (p. 212)

53. Polycythemia vera (p. 206)

54. True (p. 187)

55. False (p. 187)

56. True (p. 189)

57. True (p. 189)

58. True (p. 190)

59. False (p. 190)

60. False (p. 191)

61. True (p. 190)

62. True (p. 195)

63. False (p. 195)

64. False (p. 195)

65. True (p. 198)

66. True (p. 200)

67. False (p. 200)

68. False (p. 205)

69. True (p. 207)

70. False (p. 209)

71. True (p. 211)

Answers to the case studies in chapter 9

I. 80-year-old man
   1. The requested appointment for this gentleman should be made as soon as possible, preferably today, since you are suspicious that congestive heart failure is indicated.
   2. Age is a factor.
   3. Sodium would be restricted from the diet to lessen fluid retention. Other dietary food restrictions might be identified by the physician.

II. Single woman
   1. The circulatory condition suggested by her symptoms and circumstances is hypertension. Contributing factors are her obesity, cigarette smoking, and a probable high-fat fine diet.
   2. Diagnostic procedures called for include blood pressure on three separate occasions, auscultation, ECG, and chest x-ray.
   3. Prognosis is good with proper treatment and life-style changes.

CHAPTER 10: NERVOUS SYSTEM DISEASES

Chapter Goal

To inform students of the description, etiology, signs and symptoms, diagnostic procedures, treatment, prognosis, and prevention of the most common diseases of the nervous system.

Learning Objectives

Upon successful completion of the chapter and class lecture and discussion, students will respond to the following on a written exam within the allotted class time with a minimum of ____% accuracy.

- Identify the three main divisions of the nervous system.
- Describe the basic unit of the nervous system and how it functions.
- List the causes of headaches.
- Compare the prognoses for migraine and chronic headaches.
- Compare epidural with subdural hematomas.
- Contrast concussion and contusion.
- Recall four courses of treatment for spinal cord injuries.
- Distinguish the signs and symptoms of paraplegia and quadriplegia.
- Restate the noninjury cause of hemiplegia.
- Discuss the signs and symptoms of meningitis and encephalitis.
- Recall the prognosis for brain abscess.
- Identify at least three classifications of epilepsy.
- Describe the disease process of peripheral neuritis.
- Explain the characteristic symptoms of Bell's palsy.
- Discuss cerebrovascular accident (CVA).
- Recognize the signs and symptoms of Parkinson's disease.
- Recall the etiology of multiple sclerosis.
- Discuss the appropriate treatment protocol for amyotrophic lateral sclerosis.
- Describe the progression of brain tumors.
- List at least four signs and symptoms characteristic of nervous system diseases.

Class Activities

The "Nervous System Diseases" chapter is one of the more complex to teach, mainly because the nervous system itself is so difficult for students to understand. A neurologist can be a helpful speaker, especially if given an outline similar to the one suggested in the "Introduction" chapter of this manual.

A neurologist may be willing to bring the equipment and supplies necessary to complete a neurological examination in class. If so, students will obtain a good review of the nervous system and learn from watching such a display. A neurosurgeon may offer additional information as well.

You may choose to invite a patient from one of the nervous system disease organizations listed in the appendices of the textbook. Occupational and physical therapists involved with the rehabilitation of persons suffering from neurological diseases and disorders can be additional class supports or resources for interviews or field trips.

Name_____

Test Questions

Chapter 10: Nervous System Diseases

CIRCLE THE ONE BEST ANSWER.

1. The cause of migraine headache is often
a. Stress.
b. Tumors.
c. Infected sinuses.
d. Blood flow disruption.

2. Alternative methods of treating headaches include
a. Ingestion of garlic and onion.
b. Ingestion of refined sugars and chocolate.
c. Jogging.
d. 10 hours of sleep per night

3. Bacterial meningitis
a. Is caused by a virus.
b. Affects only the dura mater.
c. Causes nuchal rigidity.
d. Is diagnosed by a biopsy.

4. Mechanisms that may produce a stroke include
a. Cerebral hemorrhage.
b. Thrombosis.
c. Embolism.
d. All of the above

5. The cause of Alzheimer's disease is thought to be
a. Old age.
b. Head injuries.
c. Autoimmune reactions.
d. Bacterial infections.

6. A recurrent, frequently incapacitating type of headache characterized by intense, throbbing pain is called
a. Migraine.
b. Contusion.
c. Concussion.
d. Epilepsy.

7. A mass of blood formed between the skull and outer membrane covering the brain is called

a. Subdural hematoma.
b. Contusion.
c. Concussion.
d. Epidural hematoma.

8. A cerebral contusion is generally caused by
a. Blood seeping from ruptured vessels in the meninges.
b. Changes in the cerebral blood flow.
c. Vasoconstriction of cerebral-cranial arterioles.
d. A blunt impact to the head of sufficient force to cause the brain to strike and rebound   from the skull.

9. The loss of voluntary muscular control and sensation on one side of the body is called
a. Paraplegia.
b. Quadriplegia.
c. Hemiplegia.
d. Agnosia.

10. Factors that determine whether paraplegia or quadriplegia results include
The location of the spinal cord injury, the type of trauma inflicted on the cord, and the severity of the trauma.
b. Whether there is brain damage.
c. Whether there is an infectious agent.
d. a and b

11. Inflammation of the three-layer membrane that surrounds the brain and spinal cord is called
a. Encephalitis.
b. Meningitis.
c. Peripheral neuritis.
d. Bell's palsy.

12. The cause of encephalitis is
a. Bacterial.
b. Viral.
c. Pulmonary infections.
d. Cranial trauma.

13. A collection of pus usually found in the cerebellum or the frontal or temporal lobes of the cerebrum is known as
a. Encephalitis.
b. Epilepsy.
c. Organic brain syndrome.
d. Brain abscess.

14. A chronic brain disorder characterized by recurring attacks of abnormal sensory, motor, and psychological activity is called
a. Encephalitis.
b. Epilepsy.
c. Meningitis.

78

d. Brain abscess.

15. Prevention of epilepsy includes
a. Avoidance of certain foods and prompt treatment of cardiac problems.
b. Avoidance of head injuries and prompt treatment of brain infections.
c. Prompt treatment of nutritional deficiencies.
d. None of the above

16. A noninflammatory degeneration of the nerves supplying the muscles of the extremities is known as
a. Peripheral neuritis.
b. Cerebrovascular accident.
c. Transient ischemic attacks.
d. Parkinson's disease.

17. Bell's palsy is a
a. Clinical syndrome marked by the sudden impairment of consciousness.
b. Temporary, often recurring series of episodes of impaired neurologic activity.
c. Paralysis of the muscles on one side of the face due to disease of the facial nerve.
d. Chronic brain disorder characterized by recurring attacks of abnormal motor activity.

18. The following may be etiologic factors of stroke
a. Hemorrhage, embolism, and thrombosis.
b. Embolism and alcohol toxicity.
c. Thrombosis and alcohol toxicity.
d. Alcohol toxicity and nutritional deficiencies.

19. "Little strokes" are called
a. Seizures.
b. Epilepsy.
c. Strokes.
d. Transient ischemic attacks.

20. A type of chronic organic brain syndrome characterized by the death of neurons in the cerebral cortex and their replacement by microscopic "plaques" is called
a. Epilepsy.
b. Amyotrophic lateral sclerosis.
c. Alzheimer's disease.
d. Parkinson's disease.

21. A chronic nervous system disease characterized by progressive muscle rigidity and involuntary tremors is called
a. Amyotrophic lateral sclerosis.
b. Alzheimer's disease.
c. Parkinson's disease.
d. Multiple sclerosis.

22. A chronic progressive nervous disease characterized by the destruction of the myelin sheath is called
a. Amyotrophic lateral sclerosis.
b. Alzheimer's disease.
c. Parkinson's disease.
d. Multiple sclerosis.

23. Symptoms of amyotrophic lateral sclerosis include
a. Involuntary muscular contractions and weakness.
b. Muscular atrophy and problems with speech and swallowing.
c. Muscular atrophy only.
d. a and b

EVALUATE EACH STATEMENT. WRITE A *T* FOR TRUE OR AN *F* FOR FALSE ON THE LINE PROVIDED.

24. ___ Headache is caused by irritation of one or more of the pain-sensitive structures or tissues in the head and neck.

25. ___ The course of treatment for a headache is determined by the location of the headache in the head and neck.

26. ___ The prognosis for both epidural and subdural hematoma is good.

27. ___ A cerebral concussion is an immediate loss of consciousness follow by a short period of amnesia.

28. ___ A complete neurological examination is required for diagnosis of cerebral contusion.

29. ___ Much of the early treatment of quadriplegia or paraplegia is directed toward surgical intervention.

30. ___ The diagnosis of meningitis is made by performing a lumbar puncture.

31. ___ All seizures are epileptic.

32. ___ The onset of peripheral neuritis is rapid.

33. ___ Prognosis of a patient with cerebrovascular accident is determined by the extent of damage to the affected portion of brain.

34. ___ Transient ischemic attacks share a common pathophysiology with strokes and may serve as a warning of an impending cerebrovascular accident.

35. ___ Alzheimer's patients progress through three stages, ranging from mild mental impairment to an inability to care for themselves.

36. ___ The goal of Alzheimer's diagnosis is to rule out other degenerative brain diseases with similar symptoms.

37. ___ The onset of Parkinson's disease is rapid.

38. ___ The cause of multiple sclerosis is unknown, although immunologic, viral, and genetic etiologies have been proposed.

39. ___ Amyotrophic lateral sclerosis is known as Lou Gehrig's disease.

40. ___ Primary brain tumors are benign or malignant neoplasms originating within the brain.

41. ___ Secondary brain tumors are the result of metastasis of neoplasms from elsewhere in the body.

Answers

Chapter 10: Nervous System Diseases

1. d (p. 224)

2. a (p. 225)

3. c (p. 230)

4. d (p. 234)

5. c (p. 236)

6. a (p. 224)

7. d (p. 225)

8. d (p. 227)

9. c (p. 228)

10. a (p. 228)

11. b (p. 230)

12. b (p. 231)

13. d (p. 232)

14. b (p. 235)

15. b (p. 236)

16. a (p. 233)

17. c (p. 234)

18. a (p. 234)

19. d (p. 235)

20. c (p. 236)

21. c (p. 237)

22. d (p. 237)

23. d (p. 238)

24. True (p. 222)

25. False (p. 224)

26. False (p. 226)

27. True (p. 227)

28. False (p. 227)

29. False (p. 230)

30. True (p. 230)

31. False (p. 235)

32. False (p. 233)

33. True (p. 235)

34. True (p. 235)

35. True (p. 237)

36. True (p. 237)

37. False (p. 237)

38. True (p. 237)

39. True (p. 238)

40. True (p. 239)

41. True (p. 239)

Answers to the case studies in chapter 10

I. Aging mother
    1. The physician may wish to discuss Alzheimer's disease with the client.
    2. An alternative living arrangement might be necessary in order for his mother to be safe and protected from harm. A live-in arrangement or assisted-living arrangement in a retirement community could be considered.

II. 45-year-old woman
1. The diagnostic procedures a physician might order include:
    a. electromyography
    b. muscle biopsy
    c. complete medical history and exam
2. The most logical disease with these symptoms is amyotrophic lateral sclerosis (ALS).
3. Support services necessary may be home-health care, durable medical equipment, and support from the ALS Association.

CHAPTER 11: ENDOCRINE SYSTEM DISEASES

Chapter Goal

To inform students of the description, etiology, signs and symptoms, diagnostic procedures, treatment, prognosis, and prevention of the most common diseases of the endocrine system.

Learning Objectives

Upon successful completion of the chapter and class lecture and discussion, students will respond to the following on a written exam within the allotted class time with a minimum of ____% accuracy.

- Describe the two forms of hyperpituitarism.
- Discuss the signs and symptoms of hypopituitarism.
- Identify the classic symptoms of diabetes insipidus.
- Recall the cause of simple goiter.
- Explain the treatment for Hashimoto's thyroiditis.
- Recognize the signs and symptoms of hyperthyroidism.
- Compare cretinism with myxedema.
- Relate hypercalcemia to hyperparathyroidism.
- Review the classic symptoms of Cushing's syndrome.
- Recall the etiology of diabetes mellitus.
- Describe the treatment of diabetes mellitus.
- List at least four common symptoms of endocrine diseases.

Class Activities

The chapter on endocrine system diseases is a challenging one to teach, primarily because of the widespread effects the dysfunction of one endocrine gland has on the other glands. Also, diseases of the endocrine system tend to be difficult to diagnose. Symptomatology may be generalized, or even vague, and the signs and symptoms may mimic other diseases.

Speakers, however, may prove helpful in bringing the material to life. If you consider asking an endocrinologist to speak to your class, consult the "Introduction" chapter for the suggested outline for speakers.

Because diabetes mellitus is so common, you may wish to invite someone from the American Diabetes Association to speak. Another alternative is to invite a diabetic who understands the disease. However you choose to present this disease, remember to include the complications of diabetes.

An Internet search for diabetes mellitus revealed a number of interesting sources of additional information. Excite alone, one of the many available search engines, identified 23 Web sites, 12 message boards, and 11 communities related to diabetes mellitus. The authors were able to view recent news articles, clinical feature resources, medication descriptions, educational resources, legal documents, policy statements, and available books and audiovisual resources on the Internet for this disease.

Name_____

Test Questions

Chapter 11: Endocrine System Diseases

CIRCLE THE ONE BEST ANSWER.

1. Insufficient secretion of vasopressin causes
a. Diabetes insipidus.
b. Diabetes mellitus.
c. Hyperthyroidism.
d. Hypothyroidism.

2. A life-threatening complication of hypothyroidism is
a. Thyroid storm.
b. Exophthalmos.
c. Goitrogens.
d. Myxedema coma.

3. Symptoms of Cushing's syndrome include
a. Acne.
b. Moon-shaped face.
c. Grossly exaggerated head.
d. All of the above

4. Risk factors for diabetes mellitus include
a. Eating too much sugar.
b. Obesity.
c. Stress.
d. a and b

5. Diabetic retinopathy leads to
a. Ulcers.
b. Blindness.
c. Fainting.
d. Hypocalcemia.

6. Two diseases resulting from hyperfunction of the pituitary gland are
a. Simple goiter and Hashimoto's thyroiditis.
b. Grave's disease and Cushing's syndrome.
c. Cretinism and myxedema.
d. Gigantism and acromegaly.

7. Hypofunction of all of the hormones of the pituitary gland is called
a. Diabetes insipidus.
b. Gigantism.
c. Cushing's syndrome.
d. Panhypopituitarism.

8. An endocrine disease caused by insufficient secretion of vasopressin and resulting in polydipsia and polyuria is known as
a. Diabetes insipidus.
b. Gigantism.
c. Diabetes mellitus.
d. Hashimoto's thyroiditis.

9. The etiologic factors of simple goiter include
a. Dietary iodine deficiency.
b. Ingestion of goitrogens.
c. Inadequate secretion of thyroid hormones.
d. All of the above

10. An inflammatory autoimmune thyroid disease that is the leading cause of nonsimple goiter is called
a. Hypopituitarism.
b. Hashimoto's thyroiditis.
c. Graves' disease.
d. Cushing's syndrome.

11. The classic manifestations of Graves' disease are
a. Goiter, symptoms of thyrotoxicosis, ophthalmopathy, dermopathy, and nervousness.
b. Symptoms of thyrotoxicosis and ophthalmopathy only.
c. Dermopathy and nervousness only.
d. None of the above

12. Hypothyroidism appearing as a congenital condition is called
a. Hypercalcemia.
b. Myxedema.
c. Cushing's syndrome.
d. Cretinism.

13. Signs and symptoms of hyperparathyroidism include
a. Weak and brittle bones and joint pain.
b. Joint pain only.
c. Brittle bones and kidney stones only.
d. All of the above

14. Cushing's syndrome is
a. Hypersecretion of the adrenal cortex.
b. Hyposecretion of the parathyroid.
c. Hyposecretion of the thyroid.
d. Hypersecretion of the pituitary.

15. The treatment for diabetes mellitus includes a combination of
a. Hyperglycemic oral agents and analgesics.
b. Diet, exercise, and insulin.
c. Insulin and analgesics.
d. All of the above

16. Complications of diabetes mellitus include
a. Diabetic coma and insulin shock.
b. Arteriosclerotic disease and cerebrovascular accident.
c. Diabetic coma only.
d. All of the above

EVALUATE EACH STATEMENT. WRITE A *T* FOR TRUE OR AN *F* FOR FALSE ON THE LINE PROVIDED.

17. ___ The person with gigantism grows abnormally tall, although the relative proportions of the body parts and sexual development remain unaffected.

18. ___ The principal symptom of gigantism is excessive growth of the short bones of the body.

19. ___ The symptoms of acromegaly generally appear very gradually.

20. ___ Hypopituitarism is often caused by trauma to the pituitary gland or hypothalamus.

21. ___ Hormone replacement therapy is the common course of treatment for hypopituitarism.

22. ___ Vasopressin is also known as the antidiuretic hormone.

23. ___ Diabetes insipidus is a disease of the pancreas gland.

24. ___ A goiter is hypoplasia of the thyroid gland.

25. ___ The treatment goal of goiter is reduction in the size of the goiter.

26. ___ The prognosis of goiter is poor.

27. ___ The standard treatment for Hashimoto's disease is thyroid hormone replacement therapy for life.

28. ___ Hashimoto's disease can be prevented by an adequate intake of iodine.

29. ___ The course of treatment of Graves' disease depends on the affected individual's age and sex and on the severity of the case.

30. ___ Radioimmunoassay is the diagnostic procedure of choice in hyperparathyroidism.

31. ___ Treatment of hypoparathyroidism consists of lifelong vitamin D and calcium supplementation.

32. ___ The classic symptoms of Cushing's syndrome are polyuria and polydipsia.

33. ___ The treatment goal of Cushing's syndrome is to restore the concentration of serum cortisol to normal levels.

34. ___ Those with type 2 diabetes mellitus usually are overweight.

35. ___ With prompt treatment, diabetes mellitus is curable.

36. ___ A fasting plasma glucose test is the preferred way to diagnosis diabetes mellitus.

Answers

Chapter 11: Endocrine System Diseases

1. a (p. 249)

2. d (p. 255)

3. d (p. 255)

4. d (p. 256)

5. b (p. 258)

6. d (p. 247)

7. d (p. 249)

8. a (p. 249)

9. d (p. 250)

10. b (p. 251)

11. a (p. 251-252)

12. d (p. 253)

13. d (p. 254)

14. a (p. 255)

15. b (p. 257)

16. d (p. 257-258)

17. True (p. 247)

18. False (p. 247)

19. True (p. 248)

20. False (p. 249)

21. True (p. 249)

22. True (p. 249)

23. False (p. 249)

24. False (p. 250)

25. True (p. 250)

26. False (p. 250-251)

27. True (p. 252)

28. False (p. 252)

29. True (p. 252)

30. True (p. 254)

31. True (p. 254)

32. False (p. 255)

33. True (p. 255)

34. True (p. 256)

35. False (p. 257)

36. True (p. 257)

Answers to the case studies in chapter 11

I. Young woman
1. Signs and symptom suggest hyperthyroidism or Grave's disease.
2. Diagnostic procedures might include:
   a. radioimmunoassay of T_4 and T_3
   b. a thyroid radioactive iodine uptake (RAIU) test
   c. blood tests to detect antithyroid immunoglobulins
3. Other considerations include:
   a. change in sleep patterns
   b. wasting of muscle
   c. decalcification of the skeleton
   d. thickened or uneven patches of skin

II. 12-year-old boy
1. Dysfunction of the pancreas is suggested, namely diabetes mellitus.
2. A combination of diet, insulin, and exercise would be considered. Diet, insulin, and exercise are dependent upon each other, and self-management is the treatment of choice.
3. The prognosis is uncertain. A well-motivated child who follows a carefully balanced treatment regimen may delay complications for years.

CHAPTER 12: MUSCULOSKELETAL DISEASES

Chapter Goal

To inform students of the description, etiology, signs and symptoms, diagnostic procedures, treatment, prognosis, and prevention of the most common diseases of the musculoskeletal system.

Learning Objectives

Upon successful completion of the chapter and class lecture and discussion, students will respond to the following on a written exam within the allotted class time with a minimum of ____% accuracy.

- Describe three deformities of the spine.
- Identify the common cause for intervertebral disk herniation.
- Compare osteoporosis with osteomalacia.
- Recall the description for osteomyelitis.
- List at least three diagnostic procedures used specifically for determining bone disorders.
- Illustrate at least four kinds of fractures with a simple drawing.
- Compare and contrast osteoarthritis and rheumatoid arthritis.
- Describe the treatment process for bursitis and tendonitis.
- Discuss signs and symptoms of Duchenne's muscular dystrophy.
- Identify the etiology of myasthenia gravis.
- Recall the signs and symptoms of polymyositis.
- Describe the prognosis for systemic lupus erythematosus.

Class Activities

Diseases of the muscular and skeletal systems are more commonly known than many other system diseases. However, speakers can still offer additional knowledge and clarification for students. An orthopedist or physical therapist would be an appropriate guest lecturer.

Illustrations, diagrams, and x-rays are helpful for visualizing the various skeletal diseases. Please keep in mind that new treatments are found almost daily for some diseases.

Name_____

Test Questions

Chapter 12: Musculoskeletal Diseases

CIRCLE THE ONE BEST ANSWER.

1. The test to confirm an intervertebral herniated disk is the
a. Magnetic resonance imaging (MRI).
b. Computed tomography (CT) scan.
c. X-ray.
d. Straight-leg-raising test.

2. The hormone most closely associated with osteoporosis is
a. TSH.
b. ADH.
c. FSH.
d. Estrogen.

3. Diagnostic procedures for osteomyelitis include
a. Blood cultures.
b. Cultures from the site of injury.
c. Bone scan of infected area.
d. All of the above

4. A break in the bone in which a piece of the bone protrudes through the skin is a/an
a. Closed fracture.
b. Compound fracture.
c. Greenstick fracture.
d. Impacted fracture.

5. The type of fracture that is frequently found in children is
a. Closed.
b. Open.
c. Greenstick.
d. Impacted.

6. Ankylosis is the
a. Immobility of a joint.
b. Destruction of joint cartilage.
c. Over-production of synovial fluid.
d. Rupture of a synovial sac.

7. The treatment for myasthenia gravis includes
a. Non-steroidal anti-inflammatories.
b. Anticholinesterase drugs.

c. Corticosteroids.

d. b and c

8. A test performed to diagnose Systemic Lupus Erythematosus (SLE) is

a. MRI.

b. CT scan.

c. Bone marrow biopsy.

d. Anti-DNA.

9. An abnormal inward curve of a portion of the spine, commonly known as swayback, is called

a. Lordosis.

b. Kyphosis.

c. Scoliosis.

d. Cervicosis.

10. Another term for humpback is

a. Lordosis.

b. Kyphosis.

c. Scoliosis.

d. Thorocosis.

11. Treatment for deformities of the spine include

a. Physical therapy, exercise, back brace, surgery, and analgesics.

b. Exercise, back brace, and surgery only.

c. Back brace and analgesics only.

d. Surgery only.

12. Which of the following is usually the cause of a herniated intervertebral disk?

a. Insufficient bodily stores of vitamin D

b. Inadequate calcium intake

c. Malabsorption of nutrients

d. Spinal trauma from a fall or heavy lifting

13. Which of the following statements about osteoporosis is false?

a. It is a metabolic disease.

b. The total bone mass is less than expected.

c. The prognosis is excellent for osteoporosis.

d. There is no detectable abnormality of bone composition.

14. The treatment of osteoporosis includes

a. Increased dietary calcium.

b. Increased phosphate supplements.

c. Estrogen therapy.

d. All of the above

15. Defective mineralization of the bone-forming tissue is called

a. Osteoporosis.

b. Osteomalacia.

c. Osteomyelitis.

d. Paget's disease.

16. Causes of osteomalacia include
a. Insufficient bodily stores of vitamin D and intestinal malabsorption of vitamin D.
b. Bacterial infection and autoimmune factors.
c. Spinal trauma, especially vertebral.
d. b and c

17. An infection of bone-forming tissue characterized by inflammation, edema, and circulatory congestion of the bone marrow is known as
a. Osteoporosis.
b. Osteomalacia.
c. Osteomyelitis.
d. Paget's disease.

18. The most common bacterial cause of osteomyelitis is
a. The *Staphylococcus.*
b. *Mycobacterium tuberculosis.*
c. The *Streptococcus.*
d. *Proteus* organisms.

19. A chronic skeletal disease characterized by an initial phase marked by a high rate of bone turnover is called
a. Osteoporosis.
b. Osteomalacia.
c. Rickets.
d. Osteitis deformans.

20. An individual affected with Paget's disease may experience
a. Insufficient bodily stores and intestinal malabsorption of vitamin D.
b. Bacterial infection.
c. Autoimmune factors.
d. All of the above.

21. Which of the following diseases is a chronic inflammatory process of the joints and bones?
a. Osteoporosis
b. Rheumatoid arthritis
c. Osteoarthritis
d. Osteitis deformans

22. Which of the following statements about osteoarthritis is not true?
a. It results in degeneration of joint cartilage.
b. It results in hypertrophy of the surrounding bone.
c. It affects mostly weight-bearing bones.
d. None of the above

23. A chronic, systemic, inflammatory disease affecting the synovial membranes of multiple joints is called

a. Osteoporosis.

b. Rheumatoid arthritis.

c. Osteoarthritis.

d. Gout.

24. Which of the following statements is true concerning rheumatoid arthritis?

a. It can destroy cartilage and erode bone.

b. It is characterized by spontaneous remissions and unpredictable exacerbations.

c. The cause may be metabolic, renal, or both.

d. a and b

25. A chronic disorder of uric acid metabolism is

a. Rheumatoid arthritis.

b. Osteitis deformans.

c. Osteoporosis.

d. Gout.

26. Treatment of gout includes

a. Bed rest, analgesics, and low-purine diet.

b. Immobilization of the affected part.

c. Local applications of heat or cold.

d. All of the above

27. A tearing or stretching of a ligament surrounding a joint is called a

a. Sprain.

b. Strain.

c. Bursitis.

d. Tendonitis.

28. The treatment of a sprain or strain is usually

a. Surgical repair.

b. Administration of vitamin D.

c. Steroid therapy.

d. Resting and elevating the affecting part.

29. Inflammation of a thin-walled sac lined with synovial tissue is called

a. Sprains.

b. Strains.

c. Bursitis

d. Tendonitis.

30. Prevention of tendonitis includes

a. Avoidance of strenuous exercise.

b. Avoidance of contamination following trauma.

c. Ensuring adequate dietary vitamin D intake.

d. Ensuring adequate dietary calcium intake, especially milk.

31. A congenital disorder characterized by progressive bilateral wasting of skeletal muscles is called

a. Gout.
b. Polymyositis.
c. Paget's disease.
d. Duchenne's muscular dystrophy.

32. A chronic, progressive neuromuscular disease characterized by the sudden onset of drooping eyelids and double vision is called
a. Duchenne's muscular dystrophy.
b. Polymyositis.
c. Myasthenia gravis.
d. Systemic lupus erythematosus.

33. A chronic, progressive disease of connective tissue characterized by edema, inflammation, and degeneration of skeletal muscles is called
a. Duchenne's muscular dystrophy.
b. Polymyositis.
c. Paget's disease.
d. Systemic lupus erythematosus.

34. The most frequent initial manifestation of polymyositis is
a. Drooping eyelids.
b. Double vision.
c. Weakened leg and pelvis muscles.
d. Muscle weakness in hips and thighs.

35. Which of the following statements about systemic lupus erythematosus (SLE) is true?
a. SLE affects women much more than men and cannot be prevented.
b. Rashes may appear on any part of the body.
c. SLE is treated with anti-inflammatory drugs.
d. All of the above

36. The classic symptom of a bone neoplasm is
a. Bone pain.
b. Weight loss.
c. Joint deformities.
d. Muscle weakness.

EVALUATE EACH STATEMENT. WRITE A *T* FOR TRUE OR AN *F* FOR FALSE ON THE LINE PROVIDED.

37. A/an _____ is a break in the bone with no external wound in the skin.

38. A break in the bone in which there is an open wound leading down to the site of the fracture in which a piece of broken bone protrudes through the skin is a/an _____.

39. A/an _____ is a fracture in which the bone is partially bent and split.

40. A fracture in which the bone is broken or splintered into pieces, often with fragments embedded in surrounding tissue is a/an _____.

41. A/an _____ is a fracture in which the bone is broken with one end forced into the interior of the other.

Answers

Chapter 12: Musculoskeletal Diseases

1. d (p. 267)

2. d (p. 267)

3. d (p. 269)

4. b (p. 270)

5. c (p. 270)

6. a (p. 273)

7. d (p. 277)

8. d (p. 278)

9. a (p. 262)

10. b (p. 262)

11. a (p. 266)

12. d (p. 266)

13. c (p. 267-268)

14. d (p. 269)

15. b (p. 268)

16. a (p. 268)

17. c (p. 269)

18. a (p. 269)

19. d (p. 270)

20. a (p. 270)

21. c (p. 272)

22. d (p. 272)

23. b (p. 272)

24. d (p. 272-273)

25. d (p. 274)

26. d (p. 274)

27. a (p. 275)

28. d (p. 275)

29. c (p. 275)

30. a (p. 275)

31. d (p. 279)

32. c (p. 276-277)

33. b (p. 277)

34. d (p. 277)

35. d (p. 278-279)

36. a (p. 279)

37. closed fracture (p. 270-271)

38. compound or open fracture (p. 270-271)

39. greenstick fracture (p. 270-271)

40. comminuted fracture (p. 270-271)

41. impacted fracture (p. 270-271)

Answers to the case studies in chapter 12

I. Postmenopausal woman
   1. The symptoms of osteoporosis are bone pain, especially in the lower back and weight-bearing bones; spontaneous fractures; and loss of height.
   2. Diagnostic procedures include:
      a. blood tests to measure levels of phosphorus, alkaline phosphatase, total protein, albumin, and creatine

    b. urinalysis to monitor the excretion of calcium, phosphate, creatinine, and hydroxyproline

    c. x-rays

    d. bone scintiscan

    e. bone biopsy

    f. CT scan

3. Treatment depends upon the cause, but may include:

    a. increased dietary calcium, phosphate supplements, and multivitamins

    b. estrogen therapy

    c. exercise, analgesics,

    d. and muscle relaxants.

II.   Mail carrier

1. The most probable diagnosis is gout.

2. Additional information the physician might want include a medical history and physical exam. A urinalysis, laboratory tests (including ESR and WBC), and x-rays may be ordered.

3. The walking required of a postal worker places unusual stress on bones and joints. Suggest a rural route where the postman can deliver the mail via auto.

CHAPTER 13: SKIN DISEASES

Chapter Goal

To inform students of the description, etiology, signs and symptoms, diagnostic procedures, treatment, prognosis, and prevention of the more common diseases of the skin.

Learning Objectives

Upon successful completion of the chapter and class lecture and discussion, students will respond to the following on a written exam within the allotted class time with a minimum of _____% accuracy.

- Compare and contrast seborrheic dermatitis and psoriasis.
- Identify the etiology of contact and atopic dermatitis.
- Compare the life of a normal skin cell to that of a psoriatic skin cell.
- Identify the signs and symptoms of urticaria.
- Discuss the progression that occurs when a comedo becomes an acne pustule or papule.
- List at least five causes of alopecia.
- Recall the sources of infection of herpes simplex.
- Describe the etiologic process of herpes zoster.
- Restate the prognosis and prevention for impetigo.
- Compare and contrast furuncle and carbuncle.
- List the three common locations for pediculosis.
- Discuss the prevention of decubitus ulcers.
- Recall the five areas where dermatophytosis is likely to occur.
- Recall the treatment for corns and calluses.
- Identify the etiology of warts.
- Describe the signs and symptoms of discoid lupus erythematosus.
- Restate the prognosis for scleroderma.
- Name the two most common types of skin cancer.
- Identify the four types of malignant melanoma.
- Explain the treatment of diaper rash.
- List at least four common symptoms of skin diseases.

Class Activities

The study of skin diseases is best accomplished through the use of visual aids. Pictures are worth a thousand words in this chapter. Developing the skill of observation is so important in dermatology, and students will become aware of this when offered photographs and pictures of actual skin diseases.

Arranging for a dermatologist to describe the types of patients referred to them and the diagnostic procedures they use will also enhance your students' learning.

Name_____

Test Questions

Chapter 13: Skin diseases

CIRCLE THE ONE BEST ANSWER.

1. A dome-shaped or flat-topped elevated lesion, slightly reddened with intense itching
is a
a. Macule.
b. Wheal.
c. Pustule.
d. Vesicle.

2. The rash that is commonly associated with the ingestion of foods such as berries and
shellfish is
a. Urticaria.
b. Dermatitis.
c. Psoriasis.
d. Impetigo.

3. The usual cause of impetigo is
a. Carbuncle.
b. Pediculosis.
c. Mosquito bite.
d. *Streptococcus* or *Staphylococcus* bacteria.

4. Treatment for scleroderma is
a. Palliative.
b. Anti-inflammatories.
c. Radiation.
d. Corticosteroids.

5. Inflammation of the skin manifested by itching, redness, and the appearance of
various skin lesions is called
a. Psoriasis.
b. Dermatitis.
c. Acne vulgaris.
d. Fever blisters.

6. A chronic functional disease of the sebaceous glands is called
a. Seborrheic dermatitis.
b. Contact dermatitis.
c. Atopic dermatitis.
d. Psoriasis.

7. An acute inflammation caused by the direct action of various irritants on the surface of the skin is called
a. Seborrheic dermatitis.
b. Contact dermatitis.
c. Atopic dermatitis.
d. Psoriasis.

8. The best prevention of contact dermatitis is
a. Avoidance of infected persons.
b. Good oral hygiene.
c. Avoidance of stress.
d. Avoidance of known irritants.

9. A type of idiopathic dermatitis more common in infants is called
a. Contact.
b. Seborrheic.
c. Atopic.
d. Psoriasis.

10. Which of the following statements about psoriasis is not true?
a. Psoriasis is a chronic condition.
b. Psoriasis is marked by discrete pink or dull-red skin lesions.
c. Psoriasis is marked by silvery scaling.
d. Psoriasis is infectious.

11. Which of the following are possible etiologic factors of urticaria?
a. Ingestion of certain foods and insect bites
b. Inhalants and heat or cold
c. Sunlight
d. All of the above

12. A skin disease characterized by the appearance of comedos, papules, and pustules, especially during adolescence is called
a. Acne vulgaris.
b. Atopic dermatitis.
c. Urticaria.
d. Alopecia.

13. Which of the following may be treatments for alopecia?
a. No treatment and surgical autografting
b. Antipruritics
c. Androgen medication
d. a and c

14. The treatment of furuncles and carbuncles may include
a. Cleansing with soap and water, and antibiotic agents.
b. Hot, wet compresses and surgical incision and drainage.
c. None of the above
d. All of the above

15. Which of the following individuals would be at high risk to develop decubitus ulcers?
a. Patients who are immobilized
b. Patients with poor circulation
c. Unconscious patients
d. All of the above

16. Horny indurations and thickening of the stratum corneum of the skin are called
a. Dermatophytoses.
b. Corns.
c. Calluses.
d. Warts.

17. Localized hyperplasia of the stratum corneum of the skin is called
a. Dermatophytoses.
b. Corns.
c. Calluses.
d. Warts.

18. Treatment of warts includes
a. Surgical excision and keratolytic agents.
b. Metatarsal pads.
c. Cryosurgery.
d. a nd c

19. A connective tissue disorder characterized by superficial localized inflammation of the skin occurring most frequently on exposed skin surfaces is called
a. Discoid lupus erythematosus.
b. Basal cell carcinoma.
c. Malignant melanoma.
d. Dermatophytoses.

20. A progressive, chronic, systemic disease of the skin exhibiting Raynaud's phenomenon first is called
a. Scleroderma.
b. Basal cell carcinoma.
c. Dermatophytoses.
d. Malignant melanoma.

21. The goal of treatment of basal cell carcinoma and squamous cell carcinoma is to
a. Suppress the skin lesions.
b. Promote muscular function.
c. Completely eradicate the lesions.
d. Free the patient of pain.

22. Which of the following skin cancers exhibit lesions having irregular borders and a diversity of colors?
a. Malignant melanoma.
b. Basal cell carcinoma.

c. Squamous cell carcinoma.

d. Discoid lupus erythematosus.

23. An acute inflammatory eruption of highly painful vesicles on the trunk of the body is called

a. Impetigo.

b. Herpes zoster.

c. Herpes simplex.

d. Furuncles.

24. A contagious superficial skin infection marked by vesicles or bullae that become pustular is called

a. Impetigo.

b. Pediculosis.

c. Herpes simplex.

d. Furuncles.

25. Cold cores and fever blisters are caused by

a. Bacteria.

b. Viruses.

c. Fungi.

d. *Staphylococci.*

EVALUATE EACH STATEMENT. WRITE A *T* FOR TRUE OR AN *F* FOR FALSE ON THE LINE PROVIDED.

26. _____ is a fungal infection of the body.

27. _____ is a fungal infection of the scalp.

28. _____ is a maculopapular and occasionally excoriated eruption in the diaper area of infants.

Answers

Chapter 13: Skin Diseases

1. b (p. 286)

2. a (p. 287)

3. d (p. 288)

4. a (p. 298)

5. b (p. 298)

6. a (p. 298)

7. b (p. 299)

8. d (p. 299)

9. c (p. 299)

10. d (p. 287)

11. d (p. 287)

12. a (p. 288)

13. d (p. 289)

14. d (p. 291)

15. d (p. 293)

16. b (p. 296)

17. c (p. 296)

18. d (p. 297)

19. a (p. 297)

20. a (p. 298)

21. c (p. 303)

22. a (p. 303)

23. b (p. 302)

24. a (p. 291)

25. b (p. 301)

26. Tinea Corporis (p. 292)

27. Tinea capitis (p. 292)

28. Diaper rash (p. 304)

Answers to the case studies in chapter 13

I. Preschool child
    1. The signs and symptoms of impetigo are a superficial infection and itching.
    2. You should practice good hygiene and isolate the uninfected people from those infected.
    3. The cause of impetigo is *Staphylococcus* or *Streptococcus* bacterial infections.

II. 60-year-old woman
    1. The factor contributing to melanoma in this particular patient is that she plays tennis in the sun with her skin unprotected from the ultraviolet rays.
    2. The treatment indicated is surgical excision and possible chemotherapy.
    3. The prognosis is related to the level of dermal invasion and thickness of the lesion.

CHAPTER 14: EYE AND EAR DISEASES

Chapter Goal

To inform students of the description, etiology, signs and symptoms, diagnostic procedures, treatment, prognosis, and prevention of the most common diseases of the eye and ear.

Learning Objectives

Upon successful completion of the chapter and class lecture and discussion, students will respond to the following on a written exam within the allotted class time with a minimum of _____% accuracy.

- Describe four common refractive errors.
- Identify the signs and symptoms of nystagmus.
- Recall the treatment for stye.
- Discuss the prognosis for corneal abrasions.
- List the various causes of cataracts.
- Restate the prognosis and prevention for glaucoma.
- Describe the process that causes retinal detachment.
- Discuss the prevention of macular degeneration.
- Identify the signs and symptoms of conjunctivitis.
- Describe uveitis.
- Recall the signs and symptoms of blepharitis.
- Describe the treatment for impacted cerumen.
- Identify the etiology of external otitis, or swimmer's ear.
- Compare and contrast serous otitis media and suppurative otitis media.
- Define otosclerosis.
- Discuss the treatment for motion sickness.
- Recall the etiology of hearing loss.
- Restate the treatment for Ménière's disease.
- Review the prognosis and prevention of strabismus.
- List at least three common symptoms of both eye and ear diseases.

Class Activities

The "Eye and Ear Diseases" chapter can be taught as two separate subjects (the eye and the ear) with guest speakers for each segment, or in a combined format. If taught separately, an ophthalmologist would be able to discuss eye diseases very well and an otologist would be knowledgeable about diseases of the ear. Be sure to give both speakers an outline of what you expect them to cover. Consult the "Introduction" for a suggested outline for speakers.

Students' learning will also be enhanced by the use of models of the eye and the ear, as well as slides, illustrations, and diagrams, especially if many have never seen examples of eye and ear diseases.

Perhaps a visit to the office of an eye and ear specialist would be helpful, especially to emphasize the diagnostic procedures for both the eye and the ear. Other speakers might include a graduate of your program, a technician in either specialty area, or a client who suffers from one of the diseases mentioned in the text.

Name_____

Test Questions

Chapter 14: Eye and Ear Diseases

CIRCLE THE ONE BEST ANSWER.

1. A corneal abrasion is usually diagnosed by
a. Physical examination.
b. Penlight examination.
c. Fluorescein stain.
d. Culture.

2. Symptoms of otitis media would include
a. Fever and chills.
b. Nausea and vomiting.
c. Impacted cerumen with pain.
d. a and b

3. Loss of elasticity in the crystalline lens of the eye is called
a. Hyperopia.
b. Presbyopia.
c. Myopia.
d. Astigmatism.

4. The Snellen chart is used for screening
a. Eye disorders.
b. Ear disorders.
c. Endocrine disorders.
d. Nervous disorders.

5. Treatment of refractive errors of the eye includes
a. Warm compresses.
b. Contact lenses, radial keratotomy, and corrective lenses.
c. Antibiotic eye drops.
d. All of the above

6. Which of the following eye disorders is called nearsightedness?
a. Hyperopia
b. Presbyopia
c. Myopia
d. Astigmatism

7. The following may cause nystagmus:
a. Ménière's disease and multiple sclerosis.
b. Chronic visual impairment.

c. Certain drugs and alcohol abuse.

d. All of the above

8. The repetitive involuntary movement of the eye is called

a. Myopia.

b. Hyperopia.

c. Nystagmus.

d. Astigmatism.

9. A localized, purulent, inflammatory infection of sebaceous gland of the eyelid is known as

a. Hordeolum.

b. Cataract.

c. Glaucoma.

d. Retinal detachment.

10. Signs and symptoms of corneal abrasion include

a. Pain, redness, and tearing.

b. Blurring and white pupil.

c. a and b

d. Tearing only.

11. An opacity or clouding of the crystalline lens of the eye is called

a. Hordeolum.

b. Glaucoma.

c. Cataract.

d. Conjunctivitis.

12. Which of the following statements is not true for cataract?

a. The condition may be unilateral or bilateral.

b. The condition is extremely painful.

c. The gradual loss of vision is common.

d. Some patients see halos around lights.

13. The condition in which accumulating fluid pressure within the eye damages the retina and optic nerve is called

a. Cataract.

b. Glaucoma.

c. Uveitis.

d. Keratitis.

14. Which of the following diagnostic tools is used to detect intraocular pressure?

a. Snellen chart

b. Opticokinetic drum test

c. Tonometer

d. Penlight

15. Retinal detachment results in

a. A hole in the retina and abnormal fluid accumulation.

b. Complete or partial separation of the retina.

c. A *Staphylococcus* infection.

d. a and b

16. Inflammation of the mucous membrane structure that lines the inner surface of the eyelids and the anterior portion of the eyeball is called

a. Conjunctivitis.

b. Uveitis.

c. Blepharitis.

d. Keratitis.

17. The following may cause eye inflammation

a. Viruses, bacteria, and irritation from heat.

b. Irritation from chemicals and exposure to ultraviolet light.

c. None of the above

d. All of the above

18. Which of the following statements are true concerning impacted cerumen?

a. It causes permanent hearing loss.

b. It may be due to dryness and scaling.

c. A dull ring curet is used to clear the cerumen.

d. b and c

19. Which of the following describes external otitis media?

a. Pruritus and pain are common presenting problems.

b. It can be subclassified into serous or suppurative types.

c. It may be caused by rapid changes in atmospheric pressure.

d. Prevention includes prompt treatment of respiratory infections.

20. Which of the following is used to treat otitis media?

a. Antiemetics only

b. Antihistamines, antibiotics, and analgesics

c. Analgesics only

d. Antihistamines and antiemetics only

21. Formation of spongy bone, especially around the oval window, with resulting immobilization of the stapes, is known as

a. Meniere's disease.

b. External otitis.

c. Otosclerosis

d. Swimmer's ear.

22. Motion sickness is successfully treated with

a. Antihistamines

b. Antiemetics

c. Sedatives

d. All of the above

EVALUATE EACH STATEMENT. WRITE A *T* FOR TRUE OR AN *F* FOR FALSE ON THE LINE PROVIDED.

23. ___ Macular degeneration has a rapid onset.

24. ___ Drusen is symptomatic of macular degeneration.

25. ___ The most common cause of strabismus is lazy eye, or amblyopia.

26. ___ Strabismus always affects only one eye.

Answers

Chapter 14: Eye and Ear Diseases

1. c (p. 314)

2. d (p. 321)

3. b (p. 311)

4. a (p. 313)

5. b (p. 313)

6. c (p. 313)

7. d (p. 313)

8. c (p. 313)

9. a (p. 313)

10. a (p. 314)

11. c (p. 314)

12. b (p. 314-315)

13. b (p. 315)

14. c (p. 315)

15. d (p. 315-316)

16. a (p. 317)

17. d (p. 317-318)

18. d (p. 319)

19. a (p. 321)

20. b (p. 321)

21. c (p. 322)

22. d (p. 322)

23. False (p. 316)

24. True (p. 316)

25. True (p. 318)

26. False (p. 318)

Answers to the case studies in chapter 14

I. 60-year-old woman
  1. The condition indicated in this woman is cataract.
  2. Treatment options depend upon the degree of visual impairment and on the age and general health of the woman. Usually surgical extraction is followed by refractive correction.

II. Preschool girl
  1. Hearing loss in a young child could be congenital, caused by ear infection, trauma, or serious impaction of cerumen.
  2. If cause is cerumen, it should be removed. If the cause is infection, the treatment will be to administer antibiotics. Hearing loss the result of trauma may be improved by the use of hearing aids.
  3. The prognosis is excellent for a hearing loss resulting from cerumen impaction. Hearing loss from an infection usually responds well to antibiotics unless the condition is chronic. The extent of hearing loss resulting from trauma or congenital problems will determine the prognosis.

CHAPTER 15: PAIN AND ITS MANAGEMENT

Chapter Goal

To inform students of the description, purpose, pathophysiology, assessment, and treatment of pain.

Learning Objectives

Upon successful completion of the chapter and class lecture and discussion, the student will respond to the following on a written exam within the allotted class time with a minimum of _____% accuracy.

- Define pain.
- List at least four factors that influence how we experience pain.
- Discuss the purpose of pain.
- Explain the gate control theory of pain.
- Describe the pain assessment tool.
- Compare and contrast acute pain, chronic pain, and terminal pain.
- List and describe at least six types of treatment for pain.

Class Activities

Because pain is often an early symptom or one that is experienced as any disease progresses, this chapter can be taught in conjunction with any other chapter in the text. However, it may be taught as a separate unit as well.

Guest lecturers may be sought from medical societies, counseling practices, biofeedback centers, massage therapy centers, and pain clinics. The instructor must keep in mind that some people are suspect about any treatment of pain. What may be acceptable to some may repel others.

This chapter lends itself to further research by students, especially in the areas of medications, autohypnosis, relaxation, humor, laughter, play, and music. Oral reports on these interesting topics work well. Also, experienced practitioners may be willing to provide "mini sessions" for students to learn firsthand about what clients experience.

Helping students examine their preconceived notions about pain and its treatment is helpful, too. Consider asking a chronic pain sufferer to share his or her experiences with pain, and then asking students to write a report reflecting their thoughts and feelings about pain.

Name_____

Test Questions

Chapter 15: Pain and its Management

CIRCLE THE ONE BEST ANSWER.

1. Which of the following statements about pain is true?
a. Pain affects each of us during our lifetime.
b. The effects of pain may be positive as well as negative.
c. Pain is the sensation of hurting or of strong discomfort in some part of the body.
d. All of the above

2. Which of the following include the tools useful in assessing pain?
a. Place, amount, interactions, and neutralizers
b. Amount and interactions only
c. Neutralizers and place only
d. Neutralizers only

3. Chronic pain is defined as
a. Showing an increase in blood pressure and heart rate.
b. Continuous or intermittent and occurring over a period longer than 6 months.
c. A warning sign of a disturbance in physiology.
d. b and c

4. Pain therapy may include which of the following methods?
a. Medications and surgery
b. Biofeedback and autohypnosis
c. Humor, laughter, and play
d. All of the above

5. In pain therapy, TENS refers to
a. Transcutaneous electrical nerve stimulation.
b. Transmission of electrodes nerve stimulation.
c. Transfer of electricity for nerve stimulation.
d. Transverse element for nerve stimulation.

6. According to the gate control theory of pain,
a. The experience of pain is the result of the summation of the action of neurotransmitters and neuromodulators.
b. If the amount of histamine or acetylcholine exceeds the amount of endorphins at each neuron synapse, the impulse continues to the next synapse.
c. We experience pain when substances that propagate a pain impulse across each gate in a nerve pathway overpower the substances that block such an impulse.
d. All of the above

SHORT ANSWERS

7. Give your personal definition of pain.

Answers

CHAPTER 15: Pain and its Management

1. d (p. 328)

2. a (p. 330)

3. b (p. 330)

4. d (p. 331-333)

5. a (p. 332)

6. d (p. 329-330)

7. Answers will vary. (p. 328)

CHAPTER 16: THE HOLISTIC APPROACH TO DISEASE

Chapter Goal

To increase student awareness that health encompasses more than a functioning of body parts and that within a holistic approach to disease, health involves broader dimensions of a person's life including physical, spiritual, nutritional, environmental, and emotional aspects.

Learning Objectives

Upon successful completion of the chapter and class lecture and discussion, students will respond to the following on a written exam within the allotted class time with a minimum of _____% accuracy.

- Describe the connection between mind and body in relation to the disease process.
- Define holistic health care.
- Discuss personal responsibility in relation to holistic health.
- Identify at least two external and two internal environmental factors that influence our health and well-being.
- List at least four influences of personal lifestyle on holistic health.
- Describe the effects of unexpressed negative emotions on our bodies.
- Identify at least seven constructive outlets for negative emotions.
- Define stress and distress.
- Identify at least three dietary goals for the United States.
- Discuss the importance of laughter and play in holistic health.
- List at least five "playful or fun" activities.
- Compare and contrast conditional and unconditional love.
- Discuss the effects of a personal faith on a holistic lifestyle.

Class Activities

"The Holistic Approach to Disease" is a chapter some instructors will omit, either because the word holistic has a negative connotation to them or because they believe that students already understand the term. The authors challenge you, however, to include the chapter either at the beginning of your teaching of diseases to set the tone, or at the end of the class to leave students with a positive feeling about health and illness and its holistic approach.

Students often have experiences related to this chapter that they may be willing to share. Rarely has one expressed every negative emotion or not experienced stress in his or her life. It is useful when discussing this chapter to keep students "on track." For example, when students discuss stress in their lives, you may need to refocus the discussion by asking, "What influence may this have on your body? Could you become ill? What would you do if a client approached you with these complaints?"

Students can be encouraged to research holistic health further and report their findings to the class. Health practitioners who believe in and practice holistic health care may serve as speakers. Lastly, students could interview people who espouse love, friendship, laughter, or play.

Instructors will find it meaningful to teach each of the diseases chapters from a holistic approach. For example, when students are discussing the "Digestive System Diseases," specifically celiac sprue, include in your discussion how the patient might react when first diagnosed with this particular illness. Ask questions such as, "If you had to follow a special diet of no wheat, oats, barley, or rye for the remainder of your life, how would you handle it?" or "What do you think the celiac sprue client thinks or feels about the prognosis of having an increased incidence of abdominal lymphoma and carcinomas later in life?"

"The Holistic Approach to Disease" is a chapter that can be a challenge to teach, but it also can be very rewarding.

Name_____

Test Questions

Chapter 16: The Holistic Approach to Disease

CIRCLE THE ONE BEST ANSWER.

1. Holistic health is
a. A philosophy of life that relates to the whole rather than the parts.
b. An attitude and approach to life.
c. A system of care that considers the needs of the whole person.
d. All of the above

2. External environmental factors influencing personal health and well-being include
a. Genetic traits and physical characteristics.
b. Air and food.
c. Familial tendencies.
d. b and c

3. In holistic health, lifestyle is influenced by
a. Life's opportunities and personal attitudes.
b. Education and knowledge and degree of self-confidence.
c. Individual responsibilities.
d. All of the above

4. Which of the following statements is not true about stress?
a. Biological organisms require some stress in order to maintain their well-being.
b. Stress is always an indication of physical pain in the body.
c. Stress may produce pathological changes in the body.
d. The recognition of stress in one's life is key to a healthy lifestyle.

5. Personal responsibility as it relates to holistic health includes
a. The right and responsibility from birth of persons to care for themselves physically and psychologically.
b. The right of persons to observe how their bodies are functioning, and to seek medical care and treatment when needed.
c. An innate knowledge and awareness that do not need to be taught.
d. a and b

6. Laughter and play are important for experiencing holistic health because they
a. Encourage clients to think about things other than their illness.
b. Enable individuals to bond together and to express their pain or grief in the "make believe" vernacular.
c. Stimulate the release of endorphins in the body and decrease pain.
d. All of the above

122

7. Which of the following encourage holistic health and may be especially useful when a person is experiencing illness?
a. Exercise, yoga, and travel
b. Good hygiene, good nutrition, and a change in employment
c. Love, friendship, and faith
d. None of the above

Answers

Chapter 16: The Holistic Approach to Disease

1. d (p. 338)

2. d (p. 339-340)

3. d (p. 339)

4. b (p. 340)

5. d (p. 339)

6. d (p. 341-342)

7. c (p. 342-343)